Strategic Corporate Healthcare Philosophy

George O. Obikoya

Table of Content

Executive Summary	3
Introduction	5
Corporate Strategy for Healthcare Reform	8
The Corporate Paradox of Healthcare Reform	20
On Mandating Healthcare	35
Healthcare Reform and Organizational Change	46
Prospects and Challenges of Employer-Based Health Insurance	57
Healthcare Costs Kaleidoscope	68
The Line-in-Loop Corporate Healthcare Strategy	78
Employer-Sponsored Health Insurance and Healthcare Quality	91
The Medicine-Technology Dyad in Health Insurance	106
The Future of Employer-Sponsored Health Insurance	118
Conclusions	132

Executive Summary

Healthcare is at its defining moment. Plagued by crises in many countries that range from escalating costs to poor quality, and to inadequate access, and inequity, it seems to need 'radical surgery' to arrest its moribund trail. The reasons for these crises are legion, some generic, others specific to particular countries and locales. It is not that this situation is new. In fact, health systems in many countries have struggled over the years to remain viable, but seemingly to no avail. Rather, they have ended up guzzling public funds, in many instance with not much to show for it, evident in the sometimes-abysmal levels of their health quality indicators, which would make many wonder if there were no effective solutions to the healthcare delivery woes of these countries.

Given the potential for change to seem to be disruptive and for routine to appear to stabilize the status quo, that there are entrenched attitudes, even at individual levels as regards approaches to health issues is hardly surprising. Yet, that motion implies change is indubitable, as is the preference by most for it to signify that our health systems would progress rather than regress. This underlines the irony of the persistence of attitudes predicated on shaky premises, which seems to retard progress if at all any exists, in many health systems worldwide. Otherwise, it becomes inexplicable that essentially ignoring the momentum of the immense opportunities and indeed, challenges that progress in medicine and technology, as in other domains that are equally key players in the healthcare delivery dynamics has failed to have any significant impact on health services delivery other than compromise it.

The question as to whether it is time that we tried something different is therefore, redundant, considering the price of tarrying not so doing. We have bandied figures on the numbers of the uninsured and on soaring and unsustainable health spending, among others long enough and we continue to ballyhoo date solutions, regarding both of which, and that we must act now, and jettison political exigencies, and other constraints, to move our health systems forward along the path of progress, many would concur. The question is what we need to do, and how. This book attempts to answer this question. Indeed, in asserting that employer-sponsored health insurance, while not a panacea could potentially help address successfully, many of the key problems that health systems face today, as it would increasingly in the years ahead, we would no doubt unlikely soothe all nerves, literally.

Yet, this book lays bare our arguments for this position, on which eventual consensus is a realistic expectation, and goes further to discuss approaches that businesses could adopt to accomplish their healthcare services provision objectives and their important central roles in contemporary and future health systems. That firms would need to face up to these responsibilities rather than shy away from them is implicit in the realization of the benefits to them and their workers, in so doing. What are uncertain are which firms, at what rate, and to what extent would attain a realization that would likely lead them to embrace a notion that could confer on them, competitive advantage. Thus, and again, it is our expectation, that our contention in this book, might facilitate the imbuement with a culture that drives not just the flux of healthcare strategies, among firms, but also in their workforces, one upon which trust that in turn drives loyalty and commitment, crucial ingredients of enhanced productivity, predicates.

Introduction

Businesses are going to assume increasing responsibility for health services provision for their workers in the years ahead. However, and with particularly the smaller firms in countries such as the U.S., companies increasingly buckling under the financial strain of providing healthcare benefits to their workers, many no longer doing so, or requiring their workers to contribute more to their healthcare coverage, this assertion might seem bloated. Yet, firms would increasingly confront this reality, not only in the U.S., but also worldwide. The pace of adoption of the implied principles though would be, expectedly variable, and would depend on several factors, not least of which would be the desire on the part of businesses to embrace ideas such as those we develop in this book, upon which in fact their successes would likely increasingly hinge.

Even in countries that finance their health services mainly with public funds, some amount of private health insurance still exists in their health systems. It is therefore the case that many countries currently have a hybrid health financing system. However, they also have in common, health systems that are in the main, problem-ridden, inefficient, and that are ever more expensive to maintain, the services that they provide, to compound matters, often less than satisfactory. Clearly, each country would have its peculiar reasons for this undesirable state of affairs, but all need to do something to improve the situation lest their health systems and perhaps even their economies crumble in ruins. The question then is to explore the options available to solving these problems, but in doing so we would need to pay attention to the fundamental issues involved in the healthcare delivery enterprise, issues that cut across national barriers, and indeed, are sine qua non to the continuing viability of any health system.

Thus, we would consider the premise that any society requires an economy, no matter how rudimentary, to survive, and that none gets that economy going, its people sitting over a keg of wine, playing dominoes all day long. In other words, people need to work and exchange goods and services for the economy to survive, let alone thrive. In many developed countries, whose changing demographics and aging populations are creating a dearth of workers, a situation that might get worse in future, governments are starting to confront such issues headlong, increasing retirement ages, and easing up on their immigration polices, for examples. These moves underscore the central role workers play in any economy, and would continue to play at relative rates in different countries based on the human capital needs of these countries. They also highlight the need to consider issues pertaining to workers, including their health in primarily generic forms, as these issues are not unique to workers in any particular country, even if the approaches to tackling them could have varying local flavours.

In regard to workers' health therefore, our concerns should be, among others, whether they are receiving qualitative, affordable, and accessible health services, and if not, why not, and what to do about it. Central to finding answers to these questions would be where workers work to begin with, if for government or the public sector, or in private sector firms. In other words, we want to know what the employer is doing to enable workers meet their healthcare needs. No doubt, as things currently stand, neither employer-type could claim to be making this happen, and if so, why do we think that employer-sponsored healthcare coverage is the answer to the healthcare woes of workers and their families? If we accepted the fact that government in particular is not doing a great job delivering health services, as evident in the soaring healthcare spending by these governments in many countries, their health systems still faced with huge problems regardless, many would ask if at all they ought to be involved in healthcare delivery.

In a similar vein, given that, many firms are balking regarding healthcare and their health benefits costs are also on the rise, that they are also doing a good job about healthcare coverage for their employees is questionable. A major difference between the two types of employer though is that one has public funds to dig into and the other operates in a competitive global marketplace, success in which is very survival depends upon. In fact, it is this very precariousness that makes the poor performance of firms regarding their workers health now, paradoxical and that informs this book. It is also, what makes the need for government to wager regarding its continued involvement in healthcare delivery imperative. In other words, short of continuing to expend an ever-increasing percentage of the country's Gross Domestic Product (GDP) on health, which is clearly absurd, such involvement would have to predicate on improvements in the efficiency and cost-effectiveness of its healthcare delivery operations.

How these improvements would materialize government for examples, not operational in the free market, and in fact bogged down by policies that view health services through dated prisms, and which to a more or less extent, political exigencies determine, can only be conjectural. Even if in fact, it operated in the free market, the paradox of doing so with public funds would invite inevitable ruckus. On the other hand, it would be difficult if not impossible for government operations in the marketplace to match those of businesses into whose natural domains the former would have ventured. In summary, the logic of government involvement in health services would become, evidently warped, with time, given our desire to solve the problems that health systems face worldwide.

However, so would be apparent, the seeming failure of firms to recognize the important vacuum that they need to fill, in health services provision for workers, and of both to appreciate the need for freedom of choice for workers in dealing with their health issues, and indeed, for all concerned. In other words, even firms would be unable to fulfill their roles in health services provision if they did not understand and accept certain basic notions including those of choice and free market operations. Furthermore, it would not be enough to accept these fundamental notions but also important principles emanating thereof crucial to their abilities to play these roles effectively, which they need to do, not just for the sake of their workers, but also of the survivability and profitability of their organizations, and the sustenance of the wider economy in which they operate.

The aforementioned then are some of the issues we would explore in this book, to elucidate not just the key roles that businesses would play in health services provision to their workers, but also that in playing which they would be ensuring that their enterprises stand a better chance of staying afloat. We would examine the fundamental and generic issues that underlie the focus on employer-sponsored healthcare coverage that we would likely increasingly see, and how they influence the variety of issues and challenges that confront firms in health services provision for their workers and ways to address them successfully in their specific jurisdictions. Firms would have to be able to focus on and develop healthcare strategies in the years ahead. We hope that, this book would be useful in their sojourn toward achieving their stated health services provision goals.

Corporate Strategy for Healthcare Reform

The link between taxes, government spending, and the economy could be tenuous, in fact, controversial. Rubin, Orszag, and Sinai, for example contended in a 2004 study1on the effects of sustained budget deficits that estimated future deficits influence current interest rates, that smaller budget deficits lead to higher domestic private investment rates, that budget deficits result in trade deficits, and in financial and fiscal confusion, and sustaining confidence demand raising taxes. Alan Reynolds, in a CATO Institute policy analysis released shortly afterward2 disagreed with the conclusions of this study, asserting that budget deficits neither increased interest rates or trade deficits, nor reduced national savings, and were unlikely to create a financial crisis. Concerns about the potential adverse economic effects of budget deficits are not new and persist nonetheless, in particular with the increasing trend toward budget deficits by many governments, even those that hitherto had budget surpluses, $236 billion in the U.S in 20003, for example,10-year forecast estimated at $5.6 trillion 1. Indeed, many would likely consider it prudent given these circumstances to raise taxes to curtail budget deficits and improve economic growth. The economic effects of budget deficits resonate across the spectrum of activities in any country, including healthcare delivery, the most appropriate approach to financing which would likely be just as contentious as the pervasive potential effects of so doing by increasing taxes or via budget deficits, both of which we would likely increasingly witness worldwide. This is more so considering the soaring healthcare costs hence spending in many countries in recent times, 15% of GDP in the US in 2003, the highest share among the Organization for Economic Cooperation and Development (OECD) countries. US health spending is over six percent points more than the average of 8.6% in OECD countries, Switzerland and Germany, for examples, spending 11 and 11.5% of their GDP to health, respectively, Canada and France about 10%4. Additionally, demographic changes, with an increasing seniors' population in countries such as the US could in fact increase health spending, with significant implications for corporate healthcare strategy. Indeed, a January 2007 survey from Deloitte Consulting LLP and the International Society of Certified Employee Benefit Specialists showed that controlling the escalating costs of U.S. corporate healthcare benefits is the top priority for majority of benefit specialists for the seventh year in a row 5, for 91% of those polled, among their top five priorities. Eighty-two percent of benefit specialists polled indicated they were planning to redesign some or their entire healthcare and employee welfare programs, for most, cost reduction the driver but roughly, 28% listed employee recruitment, motivation, and retention as the impetus for change. No doubt, employers would continue to grapple with striking the right balance between costs curtailment and programs provision to foster recruitment and retention, among other variables that would feature more prominently in corporate healthcare strategy formulations, including more employee involvement in benefits plans payment and management. This survey actually showed that 77% of benefit specialists expect to hike employees' share of healthcare plans' costs, over 70% also planning to redesign their compensation plans, over 50%, in fact that they recently redesigned retirement programs or intend so to do. The question remains to what extent budget deficits, as in many countries these days, influence or should, such policies and plans regarding healthcare in the private sector. Tax arrangements, marginal tax rates, and the nature and extent of government spending sure influence economic growth, but in addition to indicating excessive government spending, how and to what extent, do budget deficits, actual or projected, damage the economy? What effects could this damage have on the delivery of qualitative and accessible health services and on the role of the private sector in this regard, and in which manner could it shape corporate strategy on healthcare reform? How could a preemptive strike, against projected future budget deficits via increased taxes on investors and others, for example, presumably to boost investor confidence, influence this strategy? Some would query the magnitude of the immediate effects for example of budget deficits on aggregate demand, and indeed, the value of utilizing considerations surrounding them as instruments for macroeconomic stabilization6. Yet, with the U.S budget deficit at $415 billion in 20043, expected to total around $5 trillion by 20141, hardly surprising would be concerns on government's approaches to fiscal policy including among the public, a significant proportion of who Keynesian economics deems either myopic or liquidity strapped, with a significant propensity to consume out of present disposable income, regardless. A temporary tax reduction for example, is thus, likely to have an immediate and quantitatively noteworthy effect on aggregate demand according to this viewpoint, which explains suggestions in some quarters of its benefits, which would likely stimulate interests in corporate circles, for example, on how such tax cuts could affect health-care key-player dynamics, hence determine approaches to corporate healthcare strategy. The Ricardian and Neoclassical schools of thought, the other key paradigms, on the economic effects of budget deficits offer different perspectives. None of these theories though absolutely corresponds to reality, more so given its ever-changing nature, the neoclassical view deemed by some to offer an excellent explanation of the permanent component of budget deficits, the Keynesian, the temporary, the Ricardian, dated 6, on theoretical grounds, and on oblique behavioural evidence of the bona fide, even if feeble effects of budget deficits. As earlier noted, given the skepticism of the benefits of using temporary deficits as tools for macroeconomic stabilization, should we therefore rely more on neoclassical formulation for public policy determination, with an emphasis on slashing albeit, progressively, permanent deficits simultaneously stimulating saving and capital accumulation? To what degree and how would corporate healthcare strategy depend on focus on the permanent rather than temporary components of budget deficits? Thus, would the US corporate world, for example, continue to warm up to healthcare reform as they appear set to, as soaring health costs erode profits, in a fiscal environment of even higher projected budget deficits7? The perception of the private sector in the country as being anti-healthcare reform, as it could mean either higher taxes or greater state involvement, both businesses resent, underscores the pertinence of this question, although with health costs seemingly ever increasing, that they, and how many would support such reforms, have been the subject of intense speculation lately.

With many Democratic presidential aspirants, endorsing universal healthcare coverage, and Wal-Mart aligning with the Service Employees International Union also to endorse it, the prospect of the country's corporate world being actively involved in healthcare reform does not seem that farfetched, particularly if the Democrats won the 2008 presidential or Congressional elections7. Is it any wonder that Wal-Mart and General Electric Co. for examples are keen on healthcare reforms, the former advocating universal health care coverage for all Americans by 2012? Given the annual double-digit increases in premiums in the last ten years, the average annual premium for an employer health-care plan for a four-member family, according to the National Coalition of Health Care estimates, almost $11,500, would corporate America likely discountenance healthcare reforms or would they embrace them? The US Census Bureau notes that nearly 45 million Americans lack health insurance7. Even if only one did, it is immoral many would concur to query the need to focus specifically on covering the uninsured. Yet, health economists Helen Levy of the University of Michigan's Economic Research Initiative on the Uninsured and David Meltzer of the University of Chicago argue that 'no evidence' exists that expanding coverage is cost-effective in improving health, and that other means exist that could procure more health for the funds utilized 8. Other researchers have noted that neither would expanding coverage increase overall longevity, healthcare quality, nor would it eliminate health disparities across races and socio-economic groups, or stop free-riders8. Yet, we could hardly ignore the complaints by many American firms that health costs for current and previous employees and their dependents sting the bottom line, and indeed, the consumer. For example, coverage by Ford Motor Co., in 2006, of 570,000 people at the cost of $3.5 billion, results in an additional $1,200 to the cost of each vehicle the company manufactures7. That the company still spends an added $600 per vehicle even with foreign competitors' health costs, factored, no doubt compromises its competitiveness, the effects of soaring healthcare costs not much different on other US automakers, General Motors Co. and DaimlerChrysler AG's Chrysler, for examples, and indeed, on all U.S. firms. Should they therefore not want healthcare reform, and actively participate in the exercise? The question though is how and to what extent, the answer to which Wal-Mart shareholders recently sought regarding its backing of healthcare reform, in a proposal at a June 01, 2007 meeting from the Interfaith Centre on Corporate Responsibility (ICCR), a coalition of 275 faith-based investors with assets worth about $110 billion7. Indeed, many are still unimpressed by the idea that the private sector would spearhead any healthcare reform in the US, or anywhere for that matter, in particular considering lingering questions regarding whether an employer has any responsibility for employee healthcare, and if so, to what degree. Furthermore, as in the example of California where small-group and individual health coverage is becoming out of reach as small-group premiums skyrocket, and individual-market policies coverless and demand more cost sharing, according to a recent research study by Jon Gabel and coauthors published on the Health Affairs Web site9, would companies' support for employee healthcare change focus, even flounder?

The report noted that premiums paid by employees for small-group coverage in the state rose 53 percent between 2003 and 2006, from $250 in 2003 to $382 in 2006, those for individual coverage, only 23 percent between 2002 and 2006, from $211 in 2002 to $259 in 2006, although the average actuarial value of individual coverage plummeted. For examples, individual-market policies paid, 75 and 55 percent of medical costs on average in 2003 and 2006, respectively, versus the retention in actuarial value of small-group policies, which paid for about 83 percent of medical expenses during the same period. According to this study, the analysis of the individual insurance market assumes that insurers treat a population the same as that treated in the group market, whereas California insurance law stipulates that small-group market include companies with two to fifty workers. As Gabel noted, "If you look only at premiums, individual coverage in California looks like a good deal, while small-group coverage looks increasingly expensive." He added however, that "...if you consider all out-of-pocket expenses facing policyholders, individual coverage in California is growing more unaffordable as fast as, and in fact even faster than, small-group coverage," given no statistical differences in premiums between both markets now, premiums adjusted for the financial protection particular plans offer. Compared to say 2006 when absolute premiums in small-group market were much higher than in the individual market, one cannot gainsay the need for firms to weigh strategic options given this trend. This study also showed for example that cost sharing was much higher among individual-market enrolees in 2006 than small-group-market enrolees, the average deductible in the former market, $2,136, over six times that of the latter, $348. Health Maintenance Organizations (HMOs,) which hardly ever feature deductibles, constituted almost half (44.5 percent) of all California small-group enrolment that year, but just 28 percent of the individual market, versus 37 percent in 2004. Gabel and his colleagues considered that coverage would be affordable if premiums and other out-of-pocket expenses were less than 8 percent of income, which even they considered might even be too high, coverage in the individual market essentially out of reach in the state for those at the median income level. These persons would spend 16.1 and 19.1 percent of their income for single coverage and for family coverage, respectively, worse still for those with incomes at the federal poverty level, who would spend 50.3 and 67.9 percent of their income for single coverage and for family coverage, respectively. Spending 3.5 percent of income on premiums and other expenses, in 2006, versus 2.7 percent in 2003, coverage remains affordable for single Californians at the median income, coverage would be affordable in the state for singles median income earners with regard the small-group market. For median income earning families, keen on small-group coverage, they would spend 8.2 percent of their income, slightly higher than the study's affordability benchmark, versus in 2003, an increase from 6.7 percent of income. Single coverage for those at the poverty level in the small-group market would guzzle 11 percent of income, versus 8.5 percent in 2003. Given these figures, questions arise whether companies would increasingly favour small-group insurance, which is likelier than individual insurance to meet consumer affordability standards as employers contribute a share of premiums and benefits are more all-inclusive. Some would question, however, if they would, despite what on the surface seems to be increasing costs, not mention lower cost sharing, for examples. Would firms still support health reforms for example in this regard were states in the US to adopt the Massachusetts approach and mandate individual coverage, given the likely increased earnings most would need to meet the benchmark recommended in this study for example? Firms would also be interested to know why, as in California, for example, where the same insurers hold sway in both markets the latter have different value propositions and prices for them. Gabel and his associates' interviews with insurance executives on this subject revealed, "In the individual market, insurers, based on their marketing research, were keenly conscious of 'price points'-- psychological thresholds beyond which many potential purchasers will not buy coverage. For younger potential buyers, these price points are very low." The researchers noted for example that in the state, Blue Cross of California, with its biggest share in the individual market was more successful marketing its low-cost, low-benefit product Tonik to young, healthy males, but not similar products the insurers attempted to market to the small-group market. Would such considerations affect the inclinations of firms towards the small-group market, firms in fact, more flexible in their approaches to either market, embracing one or the other based on considerations peculiar to the firms and the environments in which they operate, or not? Would demographic variables, for example, whether the firms have a preponderance of young, middle-aged, or older workers feature in these considerations, which also highlights the issue of cost sharing, considering the seeming lack of interest in the wider society of the young and healthy to purchase health insurance? Would this factor have some bearing on the focus, or otherwise of companies on one or the other of preventive or curative medicine, or both, differentially, for different age groups? This is particularly relevant in countries such as the US with three federal agencies jointly, the Departments of Treasury, Labor and Health and Human Services recently, on December 13, 2006, releasing the final regulations addressing, among other things, the "bona fide wellness program" exception to the HIPAA non-discrimination requirements. The nondiscrimination requirements, in Section 702 of the Employee Retirement Income Security Act (ERISA) (as revised by HIPAA), in general, proscribe plan sponsors from using a health factor to discriminate under a group health plan, concerning eligibility to enrol or ascertaining premium share. With this release, the provisional rules published in 1997 and 2001, clearer, firms, which are ever more incorporating financial inducements in their wellness programs, given until July 01, 2007 to comply, would have to factor some of their health promotion and disease prevention programs are subject to further HIPAA non-discrimination rules, into consideration in formulating their healthcare strategies. Plan sponsors for example might need to alter premium discount or recompense. They might need to revisit arrangements for employees unable because of ill health to meet the program requirements, and develop novel ideas regarding their wellness incentives, yet not breaking the HIPAA law, which could attract excise taxes under Internal Revenue Code Section 4980D(a), in general, $100/ day for each day the plan fails to comply regarding each employee. Firms of course, could also inadvertently be flouting other federal and state laws, for examples, the Americans with Disabilities Act (ADA), which they would no doubt want to avoid in ensuring they comply with the HIPAA regulations. With limitations on "reward", which according to the regulations could be a discount/rebate of a premium contribution, a part/all-exclusion of deductibles, coinsurance, co-payments, or other cost-sharing initiatives, among others, and the regulations excluding programs for example one that recompenses employees for smoking cessation programs costs regardless of whether the employee stops smoking, the issues are legion. Besides that, the program cannot be more than 20% of the cost of employee-only coverage under the plan, for example, to prevent a reward/penalty so great to result essentially in coverage denial, the requirement that the program's design, to promote good health or prevent disease be reasonable raises pertinent liberty issues. Thus, the employer cannot impel it as conditional to the employee receiving reward, or design one that mandates excessive employee-time or the worker to illegality. Also as noted above, with regard the avoidance of the infringement of other laws, conflicts might arise in protecting individual liberty in the process. For example, with some wellness programs requiring or coaxing employees to reveal medical information, ostensibly to improve health and prevent/better manage illnesses, the nature of the incentive, could make potentially, such an otherwise voluntary exercise, coerced under the ADA. Demographic variables are likely to be just one potential consideration in formulating corporate healthcare strategies in the years ahead, although a key one in many developed countries whose populations are increasingly aging as the likely focus of the impending negotiations to fund retiree health between US automakers and the United Auto Workers (UAW) shows10. General Motors, Ford Motor, and Chrysler in the past few months have been looking at a deal struck between Goodyear Tire & Rubber and the United Steelworkers of America agreement late 2006, under which the former moved retiree healthcare commitments to an autonomous trust fund, and in exchange provided $1 billion to fund healthcare costs. It also agreed to invest some $500 million in manufacturing facilities that the union represents, the Goodyear fund, termed a voluntary employee beneficiary association (VEBA), deemed a likely issue at the bargaining table at contract negotiations in July 2007, a VEBA expected to reduce, radically, the competitive chasm compromising the automakers' profit-making compatibilities. These three firms alone, for example, would spend over $10 billion on health care in 2007. A VEBA, properly managed, would also provide the UAW significant starting capital to assure retiree health benefits for many years, and make it one of the country's largest health care payers, besides managing one of its biggest private investment funds. The union's enhanced status in the national health care debate thereof would be doubtless, yet a VEBA agreement prior to 2011 between UAW, Ford, and GM is unlikely due to court settlements from previous contract negotiations that preclude the firms modifying retiree health care benefits before then. Nonetheless, the above, albeit eclectic examples, show the issues, among others, that would feature in, and the innovative approaches that would characterize healthcare corporate strategies in the years ahead, contingent upon the developments in the health sector and beyond, crucial for companies to survive let alone thrive. If Ford for example, funded retiree health benefits at 60cents on the dollar, it would improve earnings by 17cents per share in 2008 and boost cash flow by $600 million, estimated JPMorgan's Himanshu

Patel10, and its earnings would keep improving by 25 cents per share in 2010, its cash flow increasing to nearly $1 billion. Similarly, GM would increase its cash flow by $600 million in 2008, by $1.6 billion in 2010, its stock value stable, its earnings up by 73 cents per share, albeit GM would need $29 billion, Ford, $12.5 billion to fund a VEBA, which they should be able to raise relatively easily.

These examples also highlight a crucial point about the involvement of firms in their employees' healthcare, that of the sustainability of the firms themselves. In other words, there would not even be jobs for employees not to mention healthcare provision were the firms to go under, literally. Yet, the firms are in a bind not becoming involved, as the unproductive or less productive workforce that would ensue would mean certain demise eventually for the firms anyway, not to mention the wider ramifications for the ability of any country's private sector being unprofitable, and indeed, falling apart, ultimately. It is this mutuality between the firms and their employees, which necessitates attention by both to the most appropriate corporate healthcare strategies, and in particular in relation to changes in the health system in the applicable local and national jurisdictions. The mutuality of the employer/employee dyad and economic performance would be imperative for either partner to appreciate the significance of a workable corporate healthcare strategy. In the broader sense, for example, the worker is unlikely exempt from the uncompensated cost shifts for example of the uninsured as passed on to everyone else, would dent workers' wallets literally, and indeed, employers', to a more or less extent too. More specifically, increasing premiums increases workers' compensation costs, compromises businesses, and is a recipe for reduced earnings, even job cuts, as the 52% premiums hike between 2000 and 2005 in the US, did, for example, even in the manufacturing sector with its track record of remarkable health coverage for its employees11. Indeed, employers might not at all offer coverage due to increasing premiums, non-elderly Americans with employer-sponsored insurance 70% and 62% in 1987 and 2005, respectively12. Yet firms cannot afford to have an unhealthy workforce, even if they paid workers less wages, although that corporate health strategy would increasingly be a delicate balancing act, costs the pivot, is not in doubt. This is more so that between the three, coverage of the health expenses of more than 1.1 million current and former union members and their dependents, costs about $12 billion annually, roughly 600,000 of the members, retirees13. Indeed, with negotiations on the VEBA solution mentioned earlier, which could cost the automakers between $60 billion to $65 billion in upfront costs starting, Chrysler commencing talks with UAW on July 20, 2007, Ford and GM will begin on July 23, 2007, the current UAW contract expiring Sept. 14, 2007, all the three automakers will seek to reduce costs. The reductions expected to $48 per hour in wages, pension, and health care costs for hourly workers, Ford currently paying $70.51, GM, $73.26, and Chrysler, $75.86, according to the companies' annual reports, underscore this point13. Employers cannot also afford to discountenance healthcare providers in the equation, as the reaction of the American Medical Association (AMA) on July 18, 2007 to planned reductions to Medicare physician payments in 2008 indicates14. According to Rebecca Patchin, an anesthesiologist and member of AMA's Board of Trustees, three-fifths of 9,000 physicians surveyed by AMA said that they would stop accepting Medicare beneficiaries if Medicare reimbursements, which means Minnesota's physicians alone will lose $75 million, scheduled for reduction by 10% in January 2008 took effect. This issue highlights the interrelatedness of the economy and healthcare mentioned earlier, the formula used to calculate reimbursement payments to physicians tied to the gross national product (GNP), hence payments fall when the economy slumps, as occurred in 2001. In fact, small increases in payments since then seem not to have rectified the problem, even with improvement in the economy. So does it, underscore the need to curtail health spending, federal efforts to rein to do so with

Medicare costs also responsible for the cuts, which has made it hard for doctors to bill relative to their own increasing costs, essentially resulting in patients turned away, with ominous ramifications for healthcare access and the economy. Indeed, such issues compromise the flexibility of any nation's economy, a crucial ingredient of growth, as workers, afraid to lose their healthcare coverage, become essentially immobile, the combination of insecurity and immobility of labor, potentially devastating for the economy, more so in our contemporary global economic climate. These issues also point to the likely increasing collaboration between employers and employees, and indeed, other healthcare stakeholders, including federal and state/provincial governments to find appropriate solutions to health reform issues in their respective jurisdictions. That the Massachusetts Legislature likely will make changes for example how much employers should contribute toward workers' health care, in late fall to a state law requiring all residents to obtain health coverage, observed state Joint Committee on Health Care Financing co-Chair Richard Moore (D), recently is instructive in this regard 15. Some have suggested hiking from 33% to 50% the amount employers must contribute to workers' health care to circumvent a $295-per-employee penalty, others, limiting to 10% of income the maximum amount residents' out-of-pocket payments under health insurance, which is different from the premiums-based limits in the current law. Many would contend these moves given the background in the country of employers currently spending over $390 billion per year on employee health insurance, annual health care cost hikes significantly surpassing the inflation rate, and incremental cost shifting via novel plan designs and more employee quota to the healthcare bill, among other tested schemes, failing to contain costs. Indeed, these problems could only further strengthen the resolve by firms to act to reduce healthcare spending, even if questions regarding the approaches to achieving this goal might defy straightforward answers for many such firms. One that few chief executive officers (CEOs) would hardly contend though is the need to examine the potential for making workers healthier, for them to become more physically active, quit smoking, lose weight, and in general, to adopt healthier life styles. In other words, firms would increasingly need to embrace the idea of process cycle analysis, which essentially comprises a thorough decomposition/exposition exercise to reveal not just the underlying causes of soaring health spending in the firm, but also the solutions to them, and of course, acting on these solutions. Focusing on the worker for example would reveal the need to promote health among employees, and to prevent diseases. Further analysis would lead up to, among others, the role of an emphasis on the population health approach for example of exploring the applications of primary, secondary, and tertiary principles in achieving the goals. Thorough decompositions would therefore, result in equally detailed expositions, which would reveal the appropriate approaches to addressing the issues involved, for example, weight loss, or quitting smoking, in particular, unforced, making compliance likelier, as is curtailing health spending. Thus, firms would be able to engage their workers, voluntarily, in primary prevention programs that would reduce smoking incidence, the number of new cases, for example, in secondary prevention to seek early and prompt treatment for smoking-related, and indeed, other health problems, and in tertiary prevention, in seeking and staying in treatment to prevent and address their complications. The process cycle analyses, which firms could designate their staff to conduct, or contract out to a consultant, would also reveal for examples, the role that healthcare information and communication technologies (healthcare ICT), could play in facilitating any of the prevention phases, and the need for collaborating with healthcare providers and health plans on ensuring the deployment of these technologies. Thus, firms would increasingly need to show keen interest in issues that would help them curtail health spending simultaneously ensuring their workers receive qualitative healthcare. In other words, corporate healthcare strategy would redefine the concept of healthcare accessibility, as being not just providing their workers health insurance, but providing them qualitative healthcare. It would become clear that focusing on the former alone would not reduce but rather would continue to increase their health spending. Firms would progressively, and like governments, embrace the principles embodies in the dual healthcare delivery objectives (DHDO), as the appropriate vision of strategy, in other words, they would aim to achieve the provision of accessible and qualitative health services to their workers, more efficiently and cost-effectively, in fact, reducing spending. They would engage in process cycle analyses on an ongoing basis, realizing the imperative of change on the transactions that characterize the processes culminating in healthcare delivery, to ensure that their conduction most efficiently and cost-effectively. Yet, like governments they would face difficult choices as those that the increasing prevalence of obesity reportedly threatening to overwhelming U.K's National Health Service (NHS) with increasing prevalence of cardiovascular disease and diabetes, have led to some requesting the country to have a 'fat' tax16.

The suggestion by some policymakers that government should tax foods high in saturated fats to discourage consumers buying snacks that are bad for their health, hence avert health care costs has met with strong opposition from researchers from the University of Oxford, Queen's Medical Centre, Nottingham, and the South East Public Health Observatory16. The researchers constructed a model based on consumption data and elasticity values to predict the effects of extending the U.K's 17.5 percent value-added tax (VAT) to a wider variety of foods to discourage consumption of unhealthy food. They estimated the resulting changes in demand, expenditure, nutrition, and health16, using three different tax regimens: (1) taxing the principal sources of dietary saturated fat; (2) taxing foods defined as unhealthy by the SSCg3d nutrient scoring system; and (3) taxing foods in order to obtain the best health outcome. The researchers used consumption patterns and elasticity data from the National Food Survey of Great Britain, and the health effects of changing salt and fat intake, from previous meta-analyses. They found that taxing only the principal sources of dietary saturated fat such as whole milk, butter, cakes, biscuits, ice creams, and cheese, for example would unlikely reduce and could in fact increase cardiovascular deaths by 2,500 to 3,500 a year in the UK. This is because the reduction in saturated fat is offset by a rise in salt consumption (cross-price demand elasticities), with increased prevalence of ischemic heart diseases and stroke. They also found that taxing unhealthy foods, defined by SSCg3d score, which balances nutrients against calories, sugars, salt and fats, might avert around 2300 deaths per annum, primarily by reducing salt intake, and that taxing a wider range of foods could avert up to 3200 cardiovascular deaths in the UK per annum (a 1.7% reduction). This third model however, they noted also would hike consumer costs by 4.6 percent, the most of the three models, and tax 44.5 percent of total food expenditure. The authors thus stressed the need to recognize that ignoring cross-elasticities of demand in taxing foodstuffs could result in unpredictable health effects, hence the need for a carefully targeted fat tax. With obesity a major public health issue in many countries, the issue of fat tax is unlikely to be far away from the view of policy makers in the public and private sectors alike. As the New York City ban on trans fats indicates for example, restrictions on food choices would likely increasingly be under consideration, underscoring the research findings above. Moreover, with such revelations as obesity having roughly the same association with chronic health conditions as does twenty years' aging, hence obesity costs far exceeding those of smoking or problem drinking, the condition would likely increasingly feature in corporate healthcare strategy considerations. With obesity associated with a 36 percent rise in inpatient and outpatient spending and a 77 percent rise in medications, versus a 21 percent increase in inpatient and outpatient spending and a 28 percent increase in medications for current smokers and smaller effects for problem drinkers, the condition deserves attention. Furthermore, with an estimated 3million Medicare beneficiaries eligible in 2007 for bariatric surgery under current Medicare policy, obesity is clearly an urgent public health issue, which firms cannot afford to ignore17. Along with smoking and drinking, and substance abuse/ dependence, in general among others, it would be integral aspects of health policy measures that firms would increasingly take as parts of their healthcare strategies to contain costs while ensuring qualitative health services provision. Many firms have indeed, started to pursue the 'healthy employee' strategy, with a focus on employee health and well being, courting and many accomplishing labor union buy-in, and keeping their healthcare costs in check. With a significant portion of healthcare costs in many countries from preventable chronic diseases, there is no doubt that more companies would increasingly adopt the population health strategy mentioned earlier, and establish for examples, disease prevention, health promotion and wellness programs, offer incentives for healthy lifestyles, and facilitate healthcare provision and ill employees. More would also embrace choice, employee participation in decision making regarding their health, and rational service utilization, as programs such as consumer-directed health plans promote. That the Insurance Information Institute's (III) February 2005 industry forecast indicated that casualty and property insurance premiums would rise just 2.7% in 2005, down from a projected 4.3% increase in 2004 and a 9.8% increase in 2003 was good news to businesses, but the premium growth slowdown did not appear applicable to health insurance. Significantly though as III Chief Economist Robert Hartwig, noted these slowdowns in premium growth were not at the expense of insurers' financial health, but due to "increased economic growth and higher demand associated with the current economic recovery17." Thus, given a similar economic climate, could we assume that similar slowdowns in health insurance premium growths would not compromise insurers' bottom lines, or could we not? Health insurance costs continue to plague businesses evidently, and many continue to seek the best ways to keep these costs down. The health insurance industry is also becoming increasingly involved in controlling the skyrocketing premiums costs. Hartford, Conn.-based Aetna, one of US' major health insurers, for example, is spearheading the development of practical products, tools, and information for helping businesses and their employees achieve this goal via its Aetna HealthFund® consumer-directed product suite, which provides businesses and consumers with crucial health-care decision-making information17. Its Aetna Navigator™, a member-only self-service web site is a "one-stop shop" for members seeking access to a variety of health-related tools and information to facilitate rational decision making on health matters. Aetna Navigator has for example, Health A to Z and Aetna InteliHealth, two of the industry's most advanced consumer-oriented sources for health information. It also has a number of self-assessment tools that enable consumers gauge their personal health risk and promote healthier lifestyles, and it has a preventive care schedule for necessary health screenings, such as mammograms, eye exams, and immunizations, based on age-and gender-related national guidelines. This underscores the point made earlier of not just the important role healthcare ICT would increasingly play in controlling healthcare costs while delivering qualitative services, in short, in the achievement of the DHDO, but also of the importance of its widespread adoption by all healthcare stakeholders. The technologies would no doubt also be critical constituents of the healthcare strategy considerations of businesses progressively more. Indeed, to enhance its decision-making suite, Aetna has also introduced a potent new component, "Estimate the Cost of Care", an integrated set of interactive tools, which enable members to project the cost of various treatment options prior to even visiting their physicians. With members able to view health cost information in several key categories, the tools providing a lucid contrast of estimated average in-and out-of-network costs for prescription drugs, dental and medical procedures, and tests, doctor's office visits, and the management of specific diseases and conditions, for examples, businesses would no doubt be increasingly drawn to insurers with such value propositions. In other words, those with healthcare ICT and toolsets that would enable members realize the best value from their health benefits, a crucial aspect of controlling health spending. Besides government, employers being the largest healthcare purchasers in the US, with an employer-sponsored plan currently providing most insured Americans their healthcare, healthcare reform in the country can least afford to ignore the business sector. Employers on the other hand can also not afford to shun health reform given that they need to offer all-inclusive, competitive health benefits for staff recruitment/retention purposes, not to mention to play their part in the overall health of the economy, despite budgetary pressures and shareholder/market pressure for profitability and costs containment. The stakes could only be higher with soaring healthcare costs hence the need to contain these costs simultaneously providing qualitative and comprehensive health services, to achieve which all healthcare stakeholders need to join forces, literally. Clearly, there is need to revisit the health systems' flaws, for example of managed care, to learn lessons moving forward. Managed care's goal of optimizing service utilization some would argue has turned into a nightmare for consumers, employers, and insurers alike, what many perceived as overly price slashing, provider negotiations, cost-shifting and poor care management, among others, actually led to service over-utilization and wastage, with significant cost implications for employers, many who do not want to see that happen again. These issues are also pertinent for other countries, generically, as the desire of businesses to ensure continued profitability requires that they have a healthy and productive workforce. Yet, they cannot afford to dump money down the healthcare drain literally in the process.

References

1. Robert E. Rubin, Peter R. Orszag, and Allen Sinai, "Sustained Budget Deficits: Longer-Run U.S. Economic Performance and the Risk of Financial and Fiscal Disarray," presented at the AEA-NAEFA Joint Sessions, San Diego, January 4, 2004,www.brookings.org/dybdocroot/views/pap ers/orszag/ 20040105.pdf.

2. Reynolds A. Deficits, Interest Rates, and Taxes Myths and Realities. Cato Policy Analysis No. 517. June 29, 2004. Available at: http://www.cato.org/pubs/pas/pa517.pdf Accessed on June 17, 2007

3. Available at: http://www.commondreams.org/views04/1022-26.htm Accessed on June 17, 2007

4. Available at: http://www.oecd.org/dataoecd/15/23/34970246.pdf Accessed on June 17, 2007

5. Available at: http://www.medscape.com/viewarticle/522694 Accessed on June 17, 2007

6. Bernheim DB. A Neoclassical Perspective on Budget Deficits. Journal of Economic Perspectives—Volume 3, Number 2—Spring 1989—Pages 55-72 Available at

http://web.ebscohost.com/ehost/pdf?vid=4&hid=108&sid=38e0f2ec-1ade-4a78-b149-93265d6ae365%40sessionmgr104 Accessed on June 17, 2007

7. Available at:

http://news.yahoo.com/s/nm/20070604/us_nm/healthcare_politics_usa_dc Accessed on June 17, 2007

8. Available at: http://www.cato.org/pub_display.php?pub_id=8199 Accessed on June 17, 2007

9. Available at:

http://content.healthaffairs.org/cgi/content/abstract/hlthaff.26.4.w488 Accessed on June 30, 2007

10. Available at:

http://www.kaisernetwork.org/daily_reports/rep_index.cfm?DR_ID=46056 Accessed on July 7, 2007

11. Kaiser Family Foundation and Health Research and Educational Trust. 2006. Employer Health Benefits 2006: Annual Survey. Washington DC: Kaiser Family Foundation. Reber, Sarah and Laura Tyson. 2004. Rising Health Insurance Costs Slow Job Growth and Reduce Wages and Job Quality. Working paper.

12. U.S. Census Bureau. 2006. Income, poverty, and health insurance coverage in the United States: 2005. Current Population Reports (August).

13. Available at:

http://www.kaisernetwork.org/daily_reports/rep_hpolicy.cfm#46373. Accessed on July 21, 2007

14. Available at: http://www.startribune.com/462/story/1311428.html Accessed on July 21, 2007

15. Available at:

http://www.boston.com/news/local/articles/2007/07/19/changes_seen_to_st ate_health_insurance_law/ Accessed on July 21, 2007

16. Mytton O, Gray A, Rayner M, Rutter, H. Could targeted food taxes improve health? J. Epidemiol. Community Health 2007 61: 689-694. Available at:
http://jech.bmj.com/cgi/content/abstract/61/8/689 Accessed on July 21, 2007

17. Sturm R. The Effects Of Obesity, Smoking, And Drinking On Medical Problems And Costs. Health Affairs, March/April 2002; 21(2): 245-253 Available at: http://content.healthaffairs.org/cgi/content/ abstract/21/2/245 Accessed on July 21, 2007

18. Available at:

owww.businessweek.com/adsections/2005/pdf/0515_insurance.pdf Accessed on July 22, 2007

The Corporate Paradox of Healthcare Reform

No healthcare system could claim to be effective without the healthcare consumer able to access health services affordably and conveniently when and where needed. Regardless of the financing system of a country's health system, barriers to care could constitute essentially lack of care. This is precisely to what the ever-increasing medical and insurance costs in some countries amount, which one could hardly gainsay with persons in such countries sometimes opting out of their insurance or holding up, even not seeking required healthcare due to escalating costs. Increasing costs would also progressively more impel action at the corporate level, not just for strategic reasons related to reducing costs, but also to fostering amity with employees and their unions, both reasons crucial to competitiveness at home and abroad. In tandem with the pervasive adverse effects on the economy of spiralling health spending in many countries these days, not to mention the social disparities resultant, developments in corporate healthcare the annual hikes in healthcare inflation in the US for example still much more than the overall inflation rate1, the need for corporate action on healthcare reform seems imperative. With the prospects of businesses curtailing mounting costs via the customary plan design changes for incremental cost shifting and more employee assistance increasingly evidently bleak, the corporate world is leaning more toward healthcare purchasing model reform. No doubt, healthcare costs would continue to drive corporate healthcare benefits strategies, but other factors are crucial too, for example, the competitive forces that in turn drive the labor market, which would make the tug between recruitment and retention and stemming healthcare inflation progressively more a delicate balancing act. This underscores the point of the underlying collaboration between all stakeholders crucial to any efforts at healthcare reform. Many large firms, about a quarter, according to a recent survey that the Human Capital Practice of Deloitte Consulting LLP and the Deloitte Centre For Health Solutions conducted 1, now propose some type of consumer-driven health plan (CDHP), and even more see CDHPs as the most effective way to control costs simultaneously maintaining care quality. With cost increases for CDHPs according to this survey averaging only 2.6% versus up to 8% for other plan designs, and almost 70% of respondents contemplating a CDHP as an alternative or substitute for conventional health plans in another five years, the era of corporate interests in fostering healthy lifestyles and rational healthcare purchasing decisions among employees is indeed, here. This involvement, however, brings issues of individual liberty to the fore, among others. In other words, many would wonder what the nature and extent of corporate involvement in promoting employee health, and where the red line, literally that the employer should not cross in so doing, should be. Few if any would question the wisdom in firms taking initiatives for examples, establishing corporate intranet-based health information portals, creating health newsletters, organizing health fairs, workshops, and training, even individual/group therapy sessions, and inspirational talks. It would be a different matter for example, these firms, gathering openly or surreptitiously, employee health information on which regardless of performance excellence otherwise, to base promotion and reward. The collaboration that is crucial to the efficient interplay of the employer/ employee dyad would then likely simply be nonexistent with time, quickly dissipating. This means that neither would achieve the stated objectives it set out to achieve. So would they not, for example, even given the appreciation in the corporate world of the need to encourage employees to utilize more cost-effective healthcare providers, were these providers, even if they played their part in improving the processes that culminate in efficient and cost-effective health services provision, the healthcare consumer did not. In other words, the corporate world would still confront a paradox, which could in fact create a wager regarding involvement or not in health reform, which would soon become evident is itself, inane, if the profound nature of the issues involved, remained essentially unexamined, these issue if indeed, unearthed from their cryptic depths to begin with. The need for rectifying the pervasive and seemingly enduring information asymmetry that characterizes the health sector for example, whose atavistic paternalistic roots even healthcare practitioners increasingly recognize have become more of a liability in contemporary service delivery, is not in doubt. Yet, crucial to achieving this goal within the context of the more inclusive dual healthcare delivery objectives (DHDO) of efficient and cost-effective healthcare delivery simultaneously curtailing, if not in fact, reducing health spending, is doing so with all stakeholders on board. It would therefore, be necessary for employees for instance to embrace the patient health education tools that their employers provide to promote healthy lifestyles and disease prevention, and those required for the disease management programs that more employees now increasingly initiate for their workers. Similarly, even if employees did acquire the information required for rational decision making on matters of their health, but did not, the tools, for example the healthcare information and communications technologies (healthcare ICT), required to interface with the healthcare providers whose improved value propositions enhanced provider competitiveness, the paradox would actually thrive. With these providers for example incorporating the use of these technologies in services delivery, which should make the providers the appropriate choices of a better informed healthcare consumer, in the first place, the lack of the corresponding technologies by the healthcare consumer to complement those the providers offer, would clearly compromise the efficiency and cost-effectiveness of care delivery. If the providers invested in electronic medical records for example, but the employees did not, in personal health records (PHR) systems, or indeed, in any healthcare ICT that would enable information exchange capable of facilitating the care delivery process and improving its quality, the achievement of neither would occur. Thus, employers also would still not achieve their health reform objectives, nor would employees, and indeed, the other healthcare stakeholders, theirs. This exemplifies the importance of resolving the paradox by all healthcare stakeholders appreciating first, its potential to derail their efforts to remove the barriers to qualitative healthcare that soaring healthcare costs, hence spending cause and from which they result, and the significance of their roles individually, and collectively, in eliminating the paradox. It would with this appreciation evident the unique perspective from which their perception of this paradox, and its accompaniments, for example, that of confronting the challenges posed by information asymmetry such as embracing a generic view of education would help with, should spring. The corporate world for example would begin to see the true nature and extent of their involvement in rectifying this information skew, and in particular, what education really should entail, and how its delivery should proceed. This would guide the infusion of corporate culture that would create the enabling milieu for the voluntary embrace of the principles upon which not just the acquisition of knowledge that would promote rational decision making on health matters by employees would predicate, but that also constitutes the underlay of employee loyalty crucial to cementing this culture. That this would not only engender a healthy workforce, with the potential to boost a company's bottom line, in addition to encouraging the retention of its workforce, but also help reduce its health spending, make considerations of these issues by firms prudent. It would be necessary for firms for example in ensuring the success of their disease management programs aimed at improving the outcomes of chronic diseases such as diabetes and asthma, which many do via a health plan or a specialty vendor to encourage the sort of collaboration between their employees and healthcare providers mentioned earlier. This is more so considering the important roles these technologies could play in the more efficient treatment and monitoring of these diseases. Firms should also be keen to provide disease management programs for a broader range of diseases, including mental illnesses, and some are indeed, offering such programs for low-backache and depression, for examples1. The tendency of at least the larger firms towards changing their health care purchasing model is no doubt not challenge-free, employee resistance and/or entitlement to coverage, the survey mentioned earlier noted as the biggest. This underscores the need for change management across board, that would lead to unforced acquiescence by the workforce of the need for the individual responsibility for health matters required for example in embracing the principles of healthy living and disease prevention, along with the technologies that would facilitate the process, which firms need to achieve their health reform goals. This is not to mention, the role that these technologies could play in facilitating the evaluation of the disease management programs, for example, that increasingly feature in the new plan purchasing models that many firms now adopt. It also highlights the importance of firms acknowledging the need to promote the collaboration among stakeholders that could make information exchange serve not just the purpose of improving the quality of healthcare delivery, and enabling the assessment of the outcomes of initiatives in clinical and pecuniary terms, but also facilitate the achievement by firms of their stated health reform objectives. In other words, firms would likely be stuck with the paradox that continue annual incremental maneuverings of their healthcare purchase models rather than embark on a comprehensive overhaul of these models. Furthermore, firms need to appreciate that healthcare information and communication technologies would play a central role in the interplay of the many components of the new models, in particular in information exchange and in data management across disparate operations and loci, administration, financial, insurance, clinical, and acquisition, for examples, increasingly for any corporate-wide healthcare transformation to succeed.

Health reform issues would increasingly require the attention of businesses worldwide as access to healthcare not to mention the provision of qualitative services to their workers, and indeed, to the public in general, portend success or failure directly or indirectly for them. In the US for example, in 2005, 15.9 percent of Americans were uninsured2. According to data released on August 29, 2006 by the Census Bureau, the number of uninsured Americans was a record 46.6 million in 2005. "The number of uninsured Americans reached an all-time high in 2005," noted Robert Greenstein, executive director of the Centre on Budget and Policy Priorities, adding, "It is sobering that 5.4 million more people lacked health insurance in 2005 than in the recession year of 2001, primarily because of the erosion of employer-based insurance." 2 Further, according to Census data, 46.6 million Americans were uninsured in 2005 up 1.3 million from 45.3 million uninsured in 2004. The percentage of the uninsured increased from 15.6 percent in 2004 to 15.9 percent in 2005. The number of uninsured children increased from 7.9 million in 2004 to 8.3 million in 2005. Even in states such as Wisconsin, which has one of the lowest rates of uninsured residents in the country, healthcare costs are increasing, by more than eight percent from 2003 to 2004, the state3, eighteenth among States in healthcare spending, its health expenditures in 2004 nearly US$39 million3. That these issues would increasingly bear on businesses and their strategies for health services provision to their employees is not in doubt, given the pervasiveness of their consequences, including the potential for an unwell, and uninsured child or family member to impact negatively on a worker's productivity, in the short, perhaps even in the long term. It is doubtful that businesses could afford to ignore for too long, if at all, research findings such as those of a 2007 AARP survey of Wisconsin residents age 18 to 64 on healthcare issues in their State4. The survey showed, among others, that 76 percent of respondents want the State to reduce the number of residents that do not have healthcare coverage and that all should contribute to the system to make this happen, and that 84% of Wisconsinites consider it important for the State to make healthcare more affordable for all residents. It also showed that 82% of felt that all Wisconsinites should have access to the same basic healthcare coverage, and that more than half of respondents would vote for a candidate that supported this goal. That, firms in this state, for example, would enhance their social standing, crucial to survival, and profitability, appreciating the residents' attitude to health services provision, and gearing their healthcare strategies toward consonance with the health reforms that the state would embark upon, is only prudent could indeed be an understatement. Yet, this state, or any other in the US, or indeed, in any other country, also would be failing its residents, profoundly, ignoring the corporate paradox in their health reform initiatives. In other words, they cannot afford to create a hostile environment for businesses to thrive either, and would need to recognize the tension businesses face embracing the health reforms simultaneously struggling to keep their businesses afloat. The paradox thus surfaces in different ways, which firms nonetheless must understand fully in order to address successfully. In the above example regarding Wisconsin, firms operating in the state would need to collaborate with its health authorities and other stakeholders to ensure the realization of the goals that each party set out to achieve to a more or less extent, at the very least. In fact, firms would increasingly need to operate in this conciliatory mode to advance their healthcare delivery strategies without conflict with other healthcare stakeholders. The point is in fact that it would be in their best interests to do so not just as part of being socially responsible, as beyond creating jobs in the community in which they operate, a firm ought to be garnering goodwill in any other legitimate way, knowing full well, the competitive edge potentially resultant, formally and/or informally. This is regardless of their primary markets being outside or mainly beyond that community. Thus, the cancellation of thousands of flights at the end of June and July 2007, by NW Airlines in the US due in part to the shortage of pilots many of whom were calling in sick, affected its clients worldwide, with the potential to compromise the carrier's patronage. In fact, this is no doubt a recipe for disaster for the carrier, recently emergent from a major financial quagmire, and it underscores the need for the firm, and every firm, for that matter, to have a clear healthcare strategy for its employees, recognizing the interplay of which with other crucial factors such as remuneration, and other benefits, among others. Jan Carlzon, a Swedish businessperson gained international recognition spearheading a financial turnaround at the Scandinavian airline, SAS, starting in 1981, predicated on customer service excellence, which he built around 'moments of truth,'5, crucial transactions at each phase of the customer use cycle, with excellence at none of the stages would be unlikely possible to achieve with a disgruntled workforce. In other words, in aiming to create a positive impression of a firm at every stage of contact by its clients with its operations, from the initial contact, through on-going support, and additional purchases, the firm would need to recognize the crucial role its employees would play in this regard. It would therefore need to take the necessary measures to ensure that they do, including paying attention to their healthcare needs. In other words, part of resolving the healthcare paradox is in firms managing human resources innovatively.

There is indeed, no paradox, viewed from the vantage point of the concealed benefits inherent in such a humanistic approach, wherein, the firm recognizes and appreciates the value of its workforce as much as it does of its clientele. Yet, that is just one perspective, as the existence of the paradox becomes not just real, but potentially crippling for a firm, operating in an environment that could essentially qualify as hostile in not just creating the paradox, or paradoxes, but also obstacles in the way of their resolution.

In the US for example, states are on the one hand keen to increase access to health services for their residents, even if that alone is sufficient to guarantee service quality is another matter, simultaneously, not authorizing, only eight states in the US did in 2006, tax credits or deductions to small employers that provide healthcare6. Even in states that did, some offered tax credits, others deductions, under varying conditions. In Idaho, employers could apply a $1,000 tax credit per employee earning an average rate of $15.50 or more per hour, and those defined as 'revenue-producing enterprises' employing persons earning an average rate of less than $15.50 per hour receive a $500 tax credit per employee6. In Kentucky, employers could apply in the first year, a tax credit of 20 percent of the first year premium, 15 percent for the second, 10 percent for the third, and 5 percent for the fifth year6. In Maine, the credit is applicable for employers that employees' dependents with health benefits, the credit limited to 20 percent of qualified expenses, and not over $125 per employee with covered dependents, whereas in Ohio, the premiums a small employer pays are fully deductible. They are also deductible in Oregon, even if no provisions in state law refer to this deduction, the state's income tax system allowing businesses to include their health insurance coverage costs as one of the 'costs of doing business' in computing taxable income. Depending on which state therefore a firm operates in, the challenges that the paradox of healthcare reform pose and its perception of the ease or otherwise of their resolutions, if possible, would certainly vary and be crucial determinants of its approaches to health reform, both within and outside its boundaries. Thus, the collaboration between businesses and the state for example, has to predicate on a mutual appreciation of the benefits accruable to both thereof, as no state would consider it responsible to drive businesses away from its borders, as businesses would probably not, to jettison willy-nilly, operational areas with potential economic viability. With motivation emanating from within the worker, and inherently linked with not just recompense but also and perhaps more importantly, job satisfaction, among others, meeting their workers' healthcare needs becomes imperative for businesses, both from the perspective of the workers and of the businesses themselves, given the link between productivity, driven by motivation, and service/product quality, hence eventually, profitability. The example of the NW Airlines pilots mentioned earlier underscores these issues, including the need for firms to conceptualize internal 'health reforms,' or put differently corporate healthcare strategy globally, in tandem with the overall motivational packages including rewards and wages, and overall job satisfaction, as a workable approach to resolving the healthcare paradox. However, firms would invariably end up being moribund were they unable to balance appropriately their interests in providing their workers and dependents with health services, and not drowning, literally, in the costs of so doing. Corporate healthcare strategy therefore, in seeking the happiness of workers, which is the theoretical underpinning of all the motivational factors, be it pecuniary rewards or various initiatives to boost job satisfaction, predicates on that of the firm's shareholders, or owners, otherwise the company could readily become extinct. A generic and all-inclusive starting point of a viable healthcare strategy, geared toward resolving the paradoxes faced by firms in their particular jurisdictions would therefore be apt, namely the pursuit of the happiness of both the workers and the shareholders/owners, which would be within the existing and evolving frameworks/events in the milieu in which the firms operate. In others words, the approach to resolving the paradox should be evolutionary, based on an understanding of the flux of the regulatory and other frameworks for examples, which could influence the nature of the strategy, not to mention developments in the health/healthcare fields, and in technology, even management and other domains that constitute the dynamic variables operational.

The point here is the need to recognize that businesses face a variety of challenges in provision of health services to their workers and their dependents, and that these challenges often present paradoxes the resolution of which equally typically poses a wager, which nonetheless need not be the case, even affirming the necessity to resolve them. Indeed, the ultimate healthcare paradox, companies wondering if health services provision is not commitment to 'corporate suicide,' the reason many firms do not offer their workers healthcare coverage, and others, for examples major US auto manufacturers such as General Motors, Ford, and DaimlerChrysler, are frantically negotiating with labor unions on ways to resolve the paradox, is arguably redundant. In other words, there should be no question about employers providing their workers benefits, including healthcare services, as elements of total remuneration packages as it is in their interests, and of their workers' to do so. It only becomes a paradox if in so doing the very existence of the company comes under threat, which in a sense is itself, redundant, since there would be no paradox if the workers considered it not in their best interests that this happens. It is debatable that it is not just stalled negotiations with labor unions over the contractual details of healthcare benefits that create the corporate existential threat, but also the obstacles that laws and regulations, among others, often spawn. Even then, there should be no paradox given that the states and provinces, or generally put, the governments that make these laws and regulations should not intend to drive these companies out of business, or hinder the establishment of others, compromising employment, worsening the economic and ultimately the health conditions of their peoples.

Given the full understanding by all stakeholders of the symbiotic interplay of the players in the healthcare delivery equation therefore, that a paradox should exist is indeed, nonsensical. Yet, it does, or more appropriately, they do. In fact, the challenges that businesses face in devising workable internal 'health reforms' in keeping with the direction of health reforms in the wider milieu in which they operate seems to be mounting in many health jurisdictions world wide, compound existing paradoxes, and creating new ones. Research has shown a link between the lack of health insurance and an increased risk of a decline in overall health, for example among adults 51 to 61 years old according to a study published in the New England Journal of Medicine in 2001[7]. Thus, it could not be in the interest of any firm that its workers lack health insurance. Indeed, studies have shown that persons without health insurance use less health care services[8, 9], and have more unmet healthcare needs[10], and those without health insurance have a higher mortality rate than those that have private insurance[11]. With demographic changes in some countries, particularly the developed countries, specifically population aging, threatening to shrink the workforce, and some of these countries rethinking retirement polices, some provinces in Canada for example removing the cap on retirement, older workers would increase. Given the various reasons, for these age groups lacking healthcare coverage and some countries' comprehensive health reform efforts to ensure late middle-aged adults[12] have healthcare coverage companies would need to align their healthcare strategies, accordingly, and be cognizant of these and other issues that could steer their own efforts in particular directions, necessarily. Still in the US, with the country's healthcare expenditures ever increasing, could it continue to fund a sizeable portion of its healthcare costs with taxpayers' money? Official figures back in 1996 showed that 61 percent of Americans received employer-sponsored health insurance, although this estimate included individuals reliant primarily on government insurance for example Medicare, employees whose employers arranged their insurance but made no contributions toward it, and government employees taxpayers funded their private coverage, according to a 1999 study[13]. The study found that 43.1 percent of the population relied chiefly on health insurance paid for by private-sector employers, 34.2 percent, on publicly funded insurance, 7.1 percent, bought theirs, and 15.6 were uninsured, and that only six states had over half the population had mainly private sector, employer-sponsored coverage. The authors concluded that by definitions of health insurance current then overemphasized the role of private employers and underrated the extent of government spending on health insurance. Fast-forward the issue and a decade that the US government continues to spend substantially on healthcare is no secret, or for that matter, that many businesses do not in fact offer their workers healthcare coverage. For example, using logistic regression models to examine Behavioural Risk Factor Surveillance System data for uninsurance from 1992 to 2001 in 47 states, Nelson et. al. (2004)14 found that overall, uninsurance rates rose in 35 states and but did not change in 12 states. The numbers increased among persons aged 30 to 49 years in 34 states, and 50 to 64 years, in 24 states, and among persons at middle and low-income levels in 39 states and 19 states, respectively, among those employed for wages in 33 states, and those self-employed in 18 states. The authors concluded that among adults aged 18–64,uninsurance rates rose in most states from 1992 through 2001, which they noted would likely worsen given the decrease in employer-sponsored health insurance, increasing healthcare costs, and state fiscal crises. So then, as a further question to that asked earlier, could the US government continue to spend more and more on health, and could businesses continue not to offer their workers healthcare coverage considering the issues raised in our discussion thus far, at the very least? Rather should companies not confront their 'healthcare paradoxes' head-on realizing what they stand to lose not so doing in our prevailing and increasingly global economy? For sure, over 159 million Americans, 62.4 percent of the nonelderly population, had healthcare coverage via employer-sponsored insurance in 2004, fewer workers and their families actually had employment-based health benefits15, employer-sponsored health coverage falling from 64.4 percent in 1994 to 62.4 percent in 2004. This is despite that for the nonelderly increasing between 1994 and 2000. Furthermore, public-sector health coverage rose to 17.5 percent of the nonelderly population in 2004, as did enrolment in Medicaid and the State Children's Health Insurance Program (SCHIP) by 1.8 million in 2004, now covering 13.4 percent of the nonelderly population, significantly more than in 1999, at 10.5 percent. Thus, public-sector healthcare coverage has increased while the reverse is true for employer-sponsored coverage, the sustainability of which trend, as we wondered earlier is questionable, which highlights the paradox of corporate healthcare wherein the idea employer-sponsored health insurance appears antithetical from a business perspective vis-à-vis developments in some states in the country, some would insist. Its merit regardless, such positions need addressed, and efforts by all involved made to create the enabling environment for collaboration between governments and businesses in these states to arrive at amicable resolutions to the paradoxes, which have translated into angst seemingly with such positions held. It is unlikely to be in the interests of the businesses concerned for example that the states are unable to maintain infrastructures such as roads and bridges, electricity grids, and sewage systems, all crucial to business operations because federal assistance is not forthcoming, as the federal government spends ever more of the country's gross domestic product (GDP) on healthcare. Thus, the issue of corporate healthcare paradox has so many dimensions that businesses would need to attend to them increasingly, not just to be able to construct the most appropriate healthcare strategy, but also to be able to engage in collaborative initiatives with other healthcare stakeholders to aid in achieving the strategic objectives. The benefits in so doing as we have seen do not only relate to those derivable from a healthy and productive workforce per se, but also, among others, those that relate to the interplay of variables within the larger economy, on which the success of their business operations depends. In short, businesses have a high stake in the survival of the employer-sponsored health insurance that some have described as akin to 'private social security,'16, and with more and more doctors now employed by healthcare organizations, which means they are also beneficiaries of employer-sponsored organizations17, and derive their livelihood from a health system that businesses essentially sustains. Thus, all healthcare stakeholders have a stake in employer-sponsored insurance in a country such as the US, hence the need for collaboration in resolving the paradoxes that are threatening its survival. Many would wish it were 'dead' though, contending that President Franklin D. Roosevelt should have pursued legislation on universal healthcare coverage after his 1932 election, the decision not to do so, paving the way for employer-sponsored health insurance. Yet, others would insist that despite its flaws, it seems the most viable way to provide healthcare coverage to Americans, given that it is unsustainable for government spending on health to keep increasing as it is, currently, and the potential for resolving the paradoxes earlier discussed and others resulting in more engagement by businesses in healthcare coverage for their workers. This is besides the potential of employer-sponsored health insurance to fit appropriately into the larger scheme of the economic and healthcare prospects of a country, generating the sort of collaboration mentioned earlier in response to a commitment to ensuring the realization of these prospects in which their stakes could be quite high.

In other words, that employer-sponsored health insurance is the correct approach to health insurance is the real corporate paradox given the conceptualizations of the prevailing intellectual zeitgeist. Thus, the paradox is in fact imaginary considering that an understanding of the fundamental issues involved and a genuine application of the accompanying principles to our re-conceptualizations of the interplay of the issues involved would erase the misperceived situation we consider paradoxical for businesses to offer health insurance to their workers. This would inspire us, as we have thus far argued to examine the options in making employer-sponsored health insurance work, which would require the acceptance by all healthcare stakeholders in ensuring that this happens. It would broaden our perspective of the idea of employers providing their workers healthcare coverage and open our minds to innovative ways to address the nagging healthcare delivery issues that confront us in every arena, including in the corporate domain. Put differently, the identification of the corporate healthcare paradoxes in a sense is an invitation to a crisis that is often the wellspring of creativity, and progress, and not necessarily just for businesses, but also for the entire health system of a country. Indeed, they could trigger new ways of looking at broader issues that are nonetheless, related to healthcare delivery and its challenges, for example, issues of liberty, and the operations of the free-market, issues that constitute the core of the political and economic challenges that every society faces, whether acknowledged or not by the society, or indeed, country. Thus, every country would need to start to examine its healthcare and indeed, other issues, from a comprehensive perspective, and to be willing to ground the solutions in the fundamentals on which our very existence as humans hinge. There is a huge debate going on in the US currently in anticipation of the 2008 presidential election on the issue of universal healthcare coverage, the same idea a Democrat president rejected about seventy years ago. Granted that a lot has happened since then and millions of Americans currently lack health insurance coverage, which itself is undesirable, the question is whether the panacea to these problems is universal healthcare coverage, if there is at all any, opponents of the clamour for this sort of coverage would argue. To be fair, it is unlikely that these opponents want the millions of Americans that currently do not have health insurance not do so. On the other hand, might it not be necessary also that these persons and everyone else could access qualitative health services, making mere access to perhaps deficient services more harmful more than helpful? Is it any wonder then that opinion on this crucial matter varies even among the Democratic Party frontrunners in the 2008 elections primaries, which party has been most vocal in advocating universal healthcare coverage in recent times? The point here is that this issue does not need any more politicizing but deliberate actions on appropriate solutions to get the country's health services working optimally. That every country has to examine its peculiar situation to find the appropriate solutions to its healthcare delivery woes is hardly debatable. What is not is whether they should also not be honest in admitting the realities of the fundamental principles of liberty and free-market operations on which our continued prosperity, indeed, survival as a species depends so sorely, and adapting these principles accordingly to their peculiar situations. Thus, businesses should prepare for indeed, if not actively advocate the establishment of employer-sponsored health insurance in those countries in which they do not currently exist, but in which they would eventually, in other words, to eschew the real 'paradox', which in fact potentially spells doom for such societies. So long as there are workers, and they are humans, these issues would remain with us until resolved, that is, until employers become active in health services provision for their workers, for the reasons given above, and many others, which make it auspicious for them, and indeed, all else to do so.

What would remain is figuring out the best ways to make such arrangements work, an exercise that would be ongoing given the inevitability of change and its ramifications for current practice. In the US, for example, in 1954, the Internal Revenue Service (IRS) chose to make employers' contributions to the purchase of health insurance for their workers not taxable as income to workers[18], employers' tax benefits, $188.5 billion annually by 2004[19], for every citizen that had employer-sponsored insurance, employer-sponsored insurance at its zenith in 2000, covering 66.8 percent of nonelderly Americans[15]. In fact, out-of-pocket spending by healthcare consumers in the country dropped from 48 percent of all health care costs in 1960 to 15% in 2000[20,21], as employer-sponsored health insurance absorbed much of the costs of healthcare provision to workers. Should
the country not therefore be looking at the reasons for the current state of affairs, for example the apparently unintended consequences of the Employee Retirement Income Security Act (ERISA) enacted in 1974, and trying to rectify them, and enhancing the positive aspects of employer-sponsored health insurance rather than writing it off altogether? Should it not be more concerned about the consequences of such rulings as that in 1990 by the Financial Accounting Standards Board (FASB), the Financial Accounting Statement No. 106 (FAS 106), that requires companies covering retired employees' health care expenses to record retiree health benefit liabilities on their financial statements in keeping with generally accepted accounting principles? In fact, this ruling dramatically reduced the assets of firms[20, 22], hence compromised share prices. Further, these firms, concerned about soaring healthcare costs in particular of health services provision to retirees, started to reexamine their retiree health benefit programs to contain and curtail costs. Indeed, there has been a decrease in the percentage of private-sector employers that offer health benefits to retirees in the country, 22% in 1997, just 13% in 2002, to early retirees (pre-65), and 13% in the same year to Medicare-eligible retirees (age 65 or older), versus 20% in 1997[22]. Incidentally, with the public sector confronting similar accounting standards and similar cost pressures, it is conceivable that the effects on access to care would be unlikely inspiring, calling the benefits of universal coverage into question. These issues also highlight the points we have been making about the efficient and cost-effective running of the health services in any country, regardless of its financing model, being what counts, and that in fact, free-market operations would likelier ensure the realization of these goals given

the legendary bureaucracy and other problems that compromise efficiency for example23. It is not accidental that one could make such an assertion. This is given the commitment of many developed countries to the New Public Management (NPM), essentially the public service operating with a private enterprise approach, described by Kaul (1997) as government moving from 'a concern to do, towards a concern to ensure that things are done,24' public sector ineptness yet glaring everywhere, today. To expect that these deficiencies would enhance health sector reform (HSR), as NPM expectedly should, as indeed one of the measures aimed at complementing a serious commitment to HSR, is instructive. It underscores the need for a thorough analysis of the issues involved in a particular jurisdiction in solving its healthcare delivery problems, rather than continue to ballyhoo 'narratives,' grand theories that lack practical validity. The point is that even developed countries can hardly afford the 'luxury' of time- wasting engaging in such exercises given not only the costs associated with such delays, in human and material terms, but also that they would still have to come back and do the correct thing to fix the problems, at invariably additional and higher costs. May be improving health services administration would help reduce the soaring healthcare costs in many countries, in the US for example, $1.9 trillion and 16 percent of the GDP in 200425, but there is no doubt though, that the private sector would need to continue to play a key role in offsetting much of the country's health expenditures. Indeed, this should apply to every other country, each though approaching the issues required to ensure the realization of the dual healthcare delivery objectives (DHDO) of the provision of accessible and qualitative health services efficiently and cost-effectively differently, based on their peculiarities. Thus, businesses have to confront the challenges they face in providing health benefits to their workers, and seek appropriate solutions to them, in collaboration with other stakeholders to ensure that market forces work in favour of this happening. In other words, their costs, in health insurance, and other initiatives should not have to create a paradox wherein they need to wager. This would probably not be in favour of the workers, as the companies would struggle to remain in business, and rather pass on the increased costs to workers, directly by increasing cost-sharing, or indirectly, by reducing wages and benefits.

There are of course no panaceas or 'narratives' for many of these challenges as their origins could sometimes be way beyond the health domain as earlier noted. Yet, there are solutions with the firms and associates determined to find and implement them, via a systematic process cycle analysis of the identified issues, singly and in tandem. Thus, it is not enough for a firm to want to avoid passing on soaring healthcare costs, slashing the costs in the first place, simply instituting disease prevention, and health promotion initiatives for its workers. It would likely be necessary also for that firm, not only to get its workers interested in these initiatives, but also to be cognizant of the associated measures such as their evaluation, how this would constitute reward, what the reward would be, and how much and at what frequency, which would make the initiatives work. It might be necessary for example to involve the workers' doctors and health plans in the monitoring exercise, for example, via a network of healthcare information and communication technologies (healthcare ICT) to which all involved have authenticated access at different levels, to enable perhaps even real time health information sharing. It might be necessary for the firm in fact to figure out which programs it needs to focus on versus others based on the demographics of its workers, for example. Firms may thus have to focus on a particular gender, or minority group, or age group, or disease type, depending on these demographics. Thus, a firm's healthcare strategy would involve eclectic considerations, with the exposition following decomposition that process cycle analysis of issues reveal being veritable starting points for initiatives that could eventually result in cost reduction, simultaneously offering its workers qualitative and accessible healthcare, essentially enabling it realize the DHDO, at the corporate level. It is therefore one thing for firms to recognize that they really should not have to face a paradox, but should accept that challenges lie ahead in their efforts to provide their workers qualitative health services at reasonable costs. That businesses would indeed, need to embrace the concept of healthcare reform, is inevitable, as this would increasingly constitute integral aspects of their well being. This means that they would need to be cognizant of government efforts at reforming the health system in their jurisdictions, and initiate efforts of their own to reform their approaches to health services provision for their workers on an ongoing basis. This is what the changes equally ongoing in the many domains, health, and non-health that impinge on the reform process, would demand. For example, the smooth operations of the free market should be their priority as much as health services provision efficiently and cost-effectively should, given the potential of the former to derail the achievement of the latter. Attention to these issues would become increasingly strategic for firms in an increasingly globalized economy, which as some would argue, would necessarily heighten competition, which might compromise profitability, or highlight differential profitability among industries, hence companies' wherewithal to provide health insurance. It would be important for firms to appreciate the importance of these disparate issues, to enable them anticipate the challenges ahead, hence to formulate and implement the appropriate healthcare strategies. This also underlines the importance of the collaboration between other agencies, in the private and public sectors, to ensure that healthcare provision to workers is equitable, accessible, affordable, and importantly too, qualitative. The disparities in health services provision that the differential market power of industries and the resultant disparities in the abilities of companies, which operate in different industries to provide health services would need ongoing attention to ensure the institution of the appropriate adjustments in collaboration with the relevant agencies. Firms would need to work out the most appropriate approaches to health services provision within the context of these potential challenges, given adherence to the fundamental principles of market operations, to facilitate the materialization of the concerted efforts of other market operators to achieve the ideals of health services provision to workers. In other words, firms, acknowledging as we have here argued, the importance of health services provision to their employees, would need to align their healthcare strategies toward a common goal. This is given that they would directly or otherwise, pay, in taxes, or other ways, for not so doing anyway, as government mobilizes resources to meet soaring healthcare bills consequent, again directly or otherwise, upon the firms not providing these services, or well enough. The point then is that society cannot afford to ignore health services, the fundamental roots of which assertion are self-evident, given our proclivity, in the main, to live rather than to die, and its evolutionary significance for us as a species. Someone therefore, has to pay for these services. Regardless of who is paying, it is only prudent that the provision is efficient and cost-effective, which require the collaboration of all healthcare stakeholders to achieve. The question then arises what the best way to achieve these two objectives is. There is doubtless no panacea in this regard, but that the pursuit of the mechanisms that would ensure their realization is rational and desirable is hardly contestable, which underscores our contention that businesses for which many in society work should engage in the enterprise of health services provision, as an integral constituent of the remuneration packages of their workers. The task of working out the most appropriate strategic formulations for businesses to do so should be a priority endeavour and should be eclectic in nature, involving for example collaboration with insurance companies, and ongoing in approach, for example with negotiations with insurance firms to devise novel and innovative premiums/coverage packages to deliver high-quality health services yet reduce costs. Examples of such novel packages include consumer-directed health plans, pay-for-performance (P4P) plans, and disease management programs. Clearly, these two ingredients, as our discussion shows, are crucial for the success of these businesses in actualizing these strategies and ensuring that they realize the objectives they aim to achieve. So is their ability to engineer change among service providers, in particular, hence health plans by extension, regarding service provision and quality that would enable the realization of their goals, for example the DHDO, accomplishing which would require the desire, will, and ability, to form a strong and effective coalition to effect bargaining power. That even large businesses would be decomposing increasingly to exploit scale economies in an increasingly globalized world, attests to the power small businesses have the potential to wield, increasingly. The challenge therefore would be in organizing and mobilizing membership to drive market forces to achieve their healthcare delivery goals. However, these efforts would need to be multi-pronged, addressing via process cycle analysis for example, the salient issues germane to achieving these goals. They would need for example, in pressing for providers to implement healthcare information and communication technologies in improving the efficiency and quality of health services to encourage the completion of the health information communication and sharing 'loop,' literally. This means that the implementation of these technologies would by providers alone would not achieve the objectives the businesses set out to achieve without patients, in this instance, workers, also having personal health records (PHR) technologies hooked up with their doctors' electronic medical records (EMR) for example. Furthermore, it would be important for these systems to hook up with others, for example those of the health plans, and insurance firms, and the regional/national health information network, to facilitate information sharing among healthcare providers, and others that require patient and other information to facilitate their ends of the transactions that together constitute healthcare delivery. These issues highlight the significance of a comprehensive conceptualization of healthcare strategy for businesses for the strategy to be successful in achieving its goals.

References

1. Available at:

http://www.deloitte.com/dtt/cda/doc/content/us_chs_red_cor_hea_costs_010 6.pdf
Accessed on June 24, 2007

2. Center on Budget and Policy Priorities, The Number of Uninsured Americans is at an All-Time High (August 2006).
Available at: www.cbpp.org/8-29-06health.htm Accessed on August 4, 2007

3. Henry J. Kaiser Family Foundation, Statehealthfacts, Available at:

www.Statehealthfacts.org Accessed on August 4, 2007

4. Health Care in Wisconsin: An AARP Survey of Residents Age 18 to 64, April 2007.

5. Carlzon, J. Moments of Truth. New York: HarperBusiness, 1987.

6. Available at:

http://www.statehealthfacts.org/comparetable.jsp?ind=379&cat=7#footnote1 Accessed on August 4, 2007

7. Baker DW, Sudano JJ, Albert JM, Borawski EA, Dor A Lack of Health Insurance and Decline in Overall Health in Late Middle Age. N Engl J Med 345:1106, October 11, 2001

8. Weissman JS, Epstein AM. Falling through the safety net: insurance status and access to health care. Baltimore: Johns Hopkins University Press, 1994.

9. No health insurance? It's enough to make you sick. Philadelphia: American College of Physicians/ American Society of Internal Medicine, 2000.

10. Ayanian JZ, Weissman JS, Schneider EC, Ginsburg JA, Zaslavsky AM. Unmet health needs of uninsured adults in the United States. JAMA 2000; 284:2061-9.

11. Sorlie PD, Johnson NJ, Backlund E, Bradham DD. Mortality in the uninsured compared with that in persons with public and private health insurance. Arch Intern Med 1994; 154:2409-16.

12. Jensen GA. Health insurance of the near elderly: a growing concern. Med Care 1998; 36:107-9.

13. Carrasquillo O, Himmelstein DU, Woolhandler S, Bor DH. A Reappraisal of Private Employers' Role in Providing Health Insurance

14. Nelson DE, Bolen J, Wells HE, Smith SM, Bland S. State Trends in Uninsurance Among Individuals Aged 18 to 64 Years: United States, 1992–2001. American Journal of Public Health 1992-1997. November 2004, Vol 94, No. 11

15. Fronstin P. Sources of health insurance and characteristics of the uninsured: analysis of the March 2005 current population survey. Issue brief. No. 287. Washington, D.C.: Employee Benefits Research Institute, 2005.
Available at: http://www.ebri.org/pdf/briefspdf/EBRI_IB_11-20051.pdf. Accessed on August 4, 2007)

16. Starr P. The social transformation of American medicine. New York: Basic Books, 1982.

17. Kletke PR, Emmons DW, Gillis KD. Current trends in physicians' practice arrangements: from owners to employees. JAMA 1996; 276:555-60.

18. Thomasson M. From sickness to health: the twentieth century development of

U.S. health insurance. Explor Econ Hist 2002; 32:233-53.

19. Sheils J, Haught R. The cost of tax-exempt health benefits in 2004. Health Aff (Millwood) 2004; Suppl Web Exclusives: W4-106–W4-112.

20. Blumenthal D. Employer-Sponsored Health Insurance in the United States: Origins and Implications. N Engl J Med 355:82, July 6, 2006 Health Policy Report

21. Igelhart JK. Changing health insurance trends. N Engl J Med 2002; 347:956-62.

22. The impact of the erosion of retiree health benefits on workers and retirees. Issue brief. No. 279. Washington, D.C.: Employee Benefits Research Institute, March 2005. Available at: http://www.ebri.org/publications/ib/index.cfm?fa=ibDisp&content_id=3497 Accessed on August 5, 2007

23. Solomon D. State, local officials face looming health-care tab. The Wall Street Journal. New York, November 23, 2005:A1

24. Kaul M. (1997). The New Public Administration: management innovation in government. Public Administration and Development. 17: 13-26.

25. Health care spending growth rate continues to decline in 2004. Press release of the Centers for Medicare and Medicaid Services, Baltimore, January 10, 2006. Available at: http://www.cms.hhs.gov/apps/media/press/release.asp?counter=1750 Accessed on August 5, 2007

On Mandating Healthcare

That employee health benefit plans could, among others, help boost morale, and employer recruitment and retention efforts, and offer tax advantages to employers, contributions usually deductible expenses, do not necessarily mean that all employers would embrace them. Indeed, it makes it unnecessary to wager if they all would. When former California Governor Gray Davis Gov. Gray Davis proposed to sign into law a new health care mandate in October 2003, sponsored by doctors, workers' unions, and patient advocacy groups, the mixed reception from businesses suggests opinions, indeed differ, on this issue1. This, the backdrop then of the proposed law, a model for other states, even the U.S federal government on health benefits provision for 41 million individuals lacking health insurance, and that it would mean coverage for over one million of the seven million uninsured in the state, 19% of whose residents were uninsured, versus 15% nationally, regardless. The law mandates employers with 200 or more employees to either support financially healthcare for workers and their families, or contribute to a new state fund for the uninsured, with effect from January 1, 2006, firms with 50 to 200 employees, to support only workers, the mandate only applicable to firms with 20 to 50 workers, with state tax credits.

State business groups worried about its cost implications, according to the California Chamber of Commerce, $7.2 billion annually, with employers paying 80% ($5.7 billion), employees, $1.5 billion1, and its potential to undercut jobs and economic upturn, and lead to an exodus of firms, more so given that health care premiums and workers' compensation costs had then recently gone up. Some firms, for example, Wal-Mart, opposed the legislation on grounds that it exempted firms with union contracts covering health care, whereas others, such as Safeway, with unionized workers supported it. Critics dismissed it as not just a new tax measure but also that it infringed a federal law preventing state regulation of health insurance that self-insured employers provide. The issues that this law generated typify the many that plague the idea of mandating firms to provide healthcare coverage to employees, the details of such a mandate notwithstanding. This means that firms would need to make important choices, based on realistic strategies within the context of a complex mix of variables, health, and non-health alike, in ever-changing health services provision and economic milieus. What for example does recent evidence of a hospital study published on June 14, 20072, that high medical payments do not always purchase high-quality patient care portend for firms in making such choices, and for healthcare provision for their workers? According to a Pennsylvania government survey of the state's 60 hospitals that carried out heart bypass surgery, on average per surgery, the best-paid hospital received about $100,000, the least-paid, below $20,000, yet, lengths of hospital stay and death rates in both did not differ significantly. In fact, death rates were higher than anticipated in two of the former group among 20 metropolitan Philadelphia hospitals. That one super-costly surgery could tilt the scales aside, the findings are telling in the context of soaring health spending by healthcare consumers, insurers, and employers, even states, and the US federal government. No doubt, it is imprudent to pay more for healthcare only to receive even less-qualitative services. Yet, these are issues that are gaining prominence in not only the US but in other countries too, developed and developing alike, and which in those that are inclined towards mandating businesses to provide healthcare, could be potential cause for a closer look at these and other issues that pose challenges to either party in the implementation of such schemes. In other words, firms are likely to be showing a keener interest in the link between service quality and costs, for example, as indeed, should, all healthcare stakeholders, with increasing pressures exerted on insurance carriers and hospitals to provide objective evidence of the value of care that they provide, and indeed, of their declared value propositions in general. Thus, not only would we likelier see firms demonstrating an interest in the nature and variety of services providers offer, for example, from the strategic perspectives of primary, secondary and tertiary prevention, but also the costs implications of these services, and measures of their quality. That central Pennsylvania's Geisinger Health System for example, proposes a 30-day warranty on its cardiac surgery attests to the direction these issues would likely head. We would also likelier see such disclosures of typically 'confidential' information, as Pennsylvania did, on hospital payments and treatment outcomes, which would make strategic decision-making by firms on healthcare benefits and related issues, for instance health reform in general more objective, hence more valid. The negotiation per hospital of pricing by commercial insurers, a key factor in the disparities in payments, that this report by the Pennsylvania Health Care Cost Containment Council, for example revealed, would also likely interest firms and the healthcare consumer at large, in particular in relation to treatment outcomes. This is more so, considering that better outcomes received less compensation in some cases, Main Line Health's Lankenau, for instance, with high success bypass surgeries rates, received on average from private insurers, $33,549, versus $80,000, other centres with worse treatment outcomes records received. Firms and their employees would be able to make informed decisions on how healthcare providers match up in pricing and treatment outcomes equipped with such information as in this survey, which could help cushion the potential adverse economic consequences on companies of healthcare provision and in particular in instances of mandatory compliance with certain health benefits provision. The evaluation of care quality and particularly relative to payments is not an exact science, and requires more research to tease out the variables involved, and their significance in the evaluation process. Firms also need to attend more to preventive care and to chronic diseases management, success in both increasingly hinged on the appropriate applications of healthcare information and communications technologies (healthcare ICT), among others, hence to promoting their use by healthcare providers and their employees. The findings of a recent study are instructive in this regard 3. The researchers conducted a systematic review of the clinical effectiveness of interventions using ICTs in the management and control of chronic diseases. They searched electronic databases for randomized clinical trials that assessed the effectiveness of ICTs minus those that included only telephone usage, and measured some clinical indicator, the researchers found that ICTs used in the detection and follow up of cardiovascular diseases yielded better clinical outcomes, reduced mortality, and lowered health services utilization. They also found systems used to improve education and social support to be effective. Without necessarily mandating the use of ICTs health services provision or among their workers, there is no doubt that such studies would be of increasing interests to firms, as would devising ways, for example, incentives, to promote the use of these technologies in healthcare by their workers and healthcare providers. Thus, firms would increasingly need an open-minded approach to health benefits provision that would transcend mere numbers-crunching to curtail costs, which could significantly determine their attitude and acquiescence or otherwise to the many internal and external health reform issues they would face, including certain jurisdictions mandating healthcare provision to employees in a variety of forms.

That even then, the issue of healthcare quality is likely to remain central to considerations by businesses and other healthcare stakeholders alike is, however, going to predicate on the appreciation by all concerned of the importance of the realization of the generic dual healthcare delivery objectives (DHDO), that is, at all levels, healthcare consumer, firm, state, even country. In the US, for example, this means re-visiting the seeming practice of recompensing providers for more rather than higher quality care, which assures the perpetration of the concept of payments not necessarily promoting better care. For example, with Medicare paying a fixed rate, in effect, though variable by location and hospital type, for a given service, say the same surgical operation, its outcome nonetheless, except perhaps problems, such as requiring longer hospitalizations translating to more payments, insurers following suit, quality would no doubt lag. Firms would for instance, have to start to pressure insurers to censure or even jettison providers that deliver substandard quality services, which itself presumes the availability and use of the appropriate quality measures to make such determinations relative to agreed benchmarks. These issues bear significantly on that of mandatory healthcare provision by companies and in particular on the nature and role of governments in this regard, even if we had consensus on the other key issues, legal, ethico-moral, and economic, among others, pertaining to such mandates. In other words, is it enough for governments to mandate companies to provide healthcare to their employees without rectifying such anomalies as the Pennsylvania survey mentioned above revealed and the issues arising thereof. Should government not be mandating the release of such information as would facilitate decision making on healthcare issues by the firms and their employees for instance, and are there larger health system issues that also require attention prior to legislating if at all, such mandates? Is it any wonder thus that the non-profit Foundation for Taxpayer and Consumer Rights (FTCR), on February 8, 2007, advocated for the board implementing Massachusetts' mandatory health insurance law to require HMOs and insurance firms to reveal their records and justify insurance prices4? There is no doubt that not only would we all, including the firms, unlikely want to see anyone not receive healthcare, but would also rather have qualitative health services that save lives and improve health and well being, at reasonable costs. Indeed, the acceptance of the principles of the DHDO means that we aim to provide such services not only more efficiently, but also more cost-effectively, curtailing excessive and avoidable healthcare costs, hence spending, still providing qualitative health services to all. It is doubtful that we would achieve these goals by mere legislative fiat.

Given some of the revelations of the survey mentioned earlier for example, simply mandating employers to provide healthcare for their employees does not look like the panacea, if there is in fact any. In other words, there is need for a comprehensive analysis of the approaches proposed to improving the much-needed coverage of employees and their families that should involve the coordinated efforts of all concerned, including not just businesses and unions, but also governments, insurers, and healthcare providers, among key healthcare delivery players. The issues on mandating health insurance for everyone as in Massachusetts, which became effective on July 1, 2007, are also pertinent for those mandating companies to provide healthcare coverage for their employees. Officials in Massachusetts indicate that over 130,000 persons, roughly one third of the uninsured in 2006, are now insured 5, although observers have noted that most signers are the poor that should have free or state-subsidized coverage, and those that must pay in coverage costs fully, mostly healthy young individuals, and not signing up, might now constitute most of the uninsured. The mandatory requirement that a business with more than ten workers provide health insurance is also creating problems for small businesses in particular. Since passed in April 2006, the state's health law has received significant support from all healthcare stakeholders including firms and insurers, despite their own different perspectives of the law. It is also noteworthy that healthcare consumers can compare plans' prices and buy whichever they choose of 42 plans that six insurers offer at the web site of Commonwealth Health Insurance Connector Authority that oversees the law. Yet, so are the results of a poll, published just a few days before the law took effect by the Harvard School of Public Health, the Kaiser Family Foundation, and the Blue Cross Blue Shield of Massachusetts Foundation. The survey showed that about two-thirds of the state's residents supported the law, but the same numbers also considered it would translate to increased taxes in the end, 50% that it would harm small businesses5. There are also concerns that the scheme would adversely affect low-wage workers who, offered plans by their employers would be unable to obtain less costly state-subsidized plans. This latter concern in particular, as do others, highlight the conceptual difficulties that mandating healthcare raises, and they are just as important as the other issues involved, if not, as being the starting point, even more so. Thus, why should firms contest the idea imposed by government, yet impose it on their workers on their own, curtailing choices? Yet, this precisely what some contend the recent United Auto Workers (UAW) with General Motors (GM) which reduces health plan choices show 6. The provisional contract would cut the number of health plans available to roughly 412,000 union members, retirees and their families as GM moves to curtail health spending, about $5 billion in 2006, for 1.1 million people, union and nonunion. The workers still would have comprehensive healthcare coverage, which would improve in some respects, the contract ratified, although their option regarding health and dental options would be limited, and they could expect higher copays and limitations on doctor visits. The new contract eliminates all dental HMOs, all except three HMOs, and all PPOs except Blue Cross Blue Shield of Michigan. Some would no doubt regard these developments, the requirement that with the HMOs provided in the contract being BCBS, Health Alliance Plan, and HealthPlus of Michigan, and the proposed transfer of workers and retirees now enrolled in other plans to BCBS PPO Traditional Care Network, some sort of mandate. The point is whether such mandate, imposed from within or outside is desirable, or in fact necessary, and if not, what options do firms have to achieve the dual healthcare delivery objectives, and have they explored them? GM's UAW workers currently pay a $10 copayment for a doctor's office visit with follow-up visits unrestricted annually, but would pay under the new contract, $25 per visit for five doctor visits annually under the Traditional Care Network plan, $25 for the other HMOs retained by GM also. Additionally, dental HMO for example customarily cover in full the expenses for cleanings, examinations and X-rays, but the patient has to make copays in traditional coverage. These limitations also raise questions such as if they could hurt smaller health plans and jeopardize competition by compromising high-quality performance, and the justifications for reducing visits/ increasing cost sharing, among others. Should the emphasis for example be on one or the other or on both slashing visits and increasing cost sharing, or should it in fact be on avoiding finding ways to reduce visits without the need to increase copays? Consider that a projected 63.5 million U.S. adults visited a doctor for a preventive health or gynaecological examination every year between 2002 and 2004, costs, about $7.8 billion per year, according to a report in the Sept. 24, 2007 issue of Archives of Internal Medicine7. 'The value of many preventive health services is well established, but the role of preventive health examinations (PHEs) (also called periodic health evaluations) for health promotion and screening of disease risk factors and subclinical illness remains controversial,' the authors noted. Should firms not be exploring how they could encourage the reduction in such PHEs if not indicated and insist workers pay for them, if they insisted on still having those evaluations considered unnecessary?

Indeed, about 70 percent of patients and physicians consider it important for patients to have an annual check-up, but major North American clinical organizations do not endorse strictly preventive general health or gynaecological examinations. Ateev Mehrotra, M.D., M.P.H., of the University of Pittsburgh School of Medicine and RAND Health, Pittsburgh, and colleagues, studied data from a nationally representative survey of office-based doctors carried out between 2002 and 2004. Doctors they randomly chose completed a one-page form that detailed visits by each of 30 randomly selected patients in a chosen reporting-week. In the more than three years of the survey, 181,173 outpatient visits occurred, 5,387, preventive health examinations, 3,026, preventive gynaecological examinations, which translates nationally to 44.4 million adults (20.9 percent of the population) having preventive health examinations and 19.4 million women (17.7 percent of adult women), preventive gynaecological examinations annually. These rates varied by region, persons in the Northeast 60 percent likelier to have a PHE more than in the West. They also vary by type of insurance the uninsured 50 percent less likely to have PHE than individuals with private insurance or Medicare. The study also found that 52.9 percent of preventive health examinations and 83.5 percent of preventive gynaecological examinations offered preventive services such as mammograms, cholesterol screening, and smoking cessation counselling, but offered only 19.9 percent of eight preventive services as opposed to other types of physician visits. Noted the authors,' for example, mammograms ordered at preventive health examinations, and preventive gynaecological examinations accounted for 22.9 percent and 44.7 percent of all mammograms, respectively'. They added. 'In contrast, of all visits with weight reduction counselling, only 8.8 percent were preventive health examinations and 1.1 percent were preventive gynaecological examinations.' Firms would likely increasingly take a cue from the conclusions of the authors that 'Preventive health examinations and preventive gynaecological examinations are among the most common reasons adults see a physician.These visits frequently include preventive services, but most preventive services are provided at other visits. These findings provide a foundation for continuing national deliberations about the use and content of preventive health examinations and preventive gynaecological examinations.' In other words, would attention to such issues not obviate the need to increase copays for example, and could it not ensure the right choice of providers by workers, and indeed, encourage quality improvement in declared value propositions by providers, hence promote competition, hence modulate prices? Thus, firms taking such decisions, as did GM to limit choice might in fact be compromising their ability to achieve the dual healthcare delivery objectives rather than otherwise, and as is in this instance, so might the union, which would assume responsibility for managing health benefits, from GM, via VEBA in 2010. There are indications of the potential to reduce the benefits under VEBA for example, if current projections turn out to be inaccurate, which underscores the point about the need to explore the options that would result in the achievement of the DHDO, which would make concerns over such reductions, redundant. We thus see the need to conceptualize the issue of mandating healthcare in broader terms, the adverse consequences of its imposition nonetheless potentially severe, coming from within or without the firm.

That the pursuit of the DHDO makes these concerns redundant hence warrants efforts at so doing is evident in a recent letter regarding GM's cost-curtailing effort from the AFL-CIO that the firm has not done enough to slash prescription drug costs7, that GM still has brand-name heartburn treatment Nexium on its approved-drug list, for example. Other firms for examples, Ford Motor and Chrysler Group, have removed or reduced coverage of the drug to promote use of its generic versions, which cost about $12 for a four-week supply, versus $49 for the brand. Ford Motor offers Nexium to its workers only they have tried lower-cost alternatives, and Chrysler could still buy Nexium, but would pay extra costs. Here again, we see another dimension of the issue of mandating healthcare that firms would increasingly factor into considerations on this matter were they to solve effectively the problems hindering the provision of qualitative health services, cost-effectively and efficiently, which are, or should be their primary objectives. With regard this case for example, AFL-CIO has been having talks with GM a conflict-of-interest issue regarding Nexium since June 2007, revolving over longtime GM board member Percy Barnevik being a retired chair of AstraZeneca, which makes Nexium. AFL-CIO's efforts to query the neutrality in these matters of health industry executives on the boards of some of the country's key, non-health-related firms, extends to other companies8, twenty others, and board members who were directors/executives of pharmaceutical or health insurance firms, are actually in the interests of both workers and the firms. GM spokesperson Michelle Bunker stressed that 'GM's board did not have any influence over any of the decision that our pharmacy benefits manager (PBM, which is Medco Health Solutions) makes regarding offerings.' However, director of University of Michigan's Centre for Value-Based Insurance Design, Mark Fendrick's observation that although PBMs created the preferred-drug lists, employers frequently change the lists to cut costs, is instructive, and highlights the need for an appreciation in full of the issues in the decisions firms make regarding every aspect of their healthcare strategy. Indeed, that AFL-CIO President John Sweeney in September 2007 requested GM Chair and CEO Rick Wagoner to stop three board members Barnevik; George Fisher, an Eli Lilly director; and Karen Katten, a former Pfizer vice-Chair 'playing any leadership role in consideration of health care matters at GM'. The real issue, though, is not who is on GM's board, but what decisions the board takes, and whether these decisions are in the firm's overall interests. In other words, even the board members would eventually realize the disfavour they do the firm taking decisions that hurt rather than help the firm. It is certainly conceivable that the time it takes for a firm's board, or its decision-making body to achieve this realization would vary, but so would the consequences of poor judgment on the firm's profitability, and indeed, survivability in the end. Thus, it would increasingly be crucial to the competitive edge of a firm to adopt appropriate healthcare strategies regardless of its board members and their perceived or real interests were firms to stay afloat, let alone thrive. Thus, it would be necessary to make a distinction between measures that seem on the surface to be in the firm's interest, but which actually are, often only and if at all, in the short term. Such decisions therefore, as limiting the options they and their workers have regarding health plans and healthcare providers, could only backfire in the long term. In short, firms should and would need to eschew mandating healthcare initiatives for whatever reason, preference for initiatives based on adequate considerations of the relevant issues, including process cycle analyses, which would further elucidate them, likely to characterize firms that would gain competitive advantage in future, and there is no gainsaying this point. Why, for example, would firms in the U.S., dismiss the fact that American adults are likelier than Europeans to receive the diagnosis of and treatment for chronic diseases, which higher rates contribute up to $150 billion to the country's yearly healthcare expenditure according to a new research9? Reported on October 02, 2007 in a Health Affairs Web Exclusive, the study noted that seniors in the United States are significantly likelier than those in Europe are, to have expensive chronic diseases, such as cancer, diabetes, and heart disease, and receive treatment for these conditions, and that Americans are almost twice as likely to be obese. The researchers, who compared 2004 data on the prevalence and treatment of diseases among adults age 50 and older in the U.S. and 10 European countries (Austria, Denmark, France, Germany, Greece, Italy, Netherlands, Spain, Sweden, and Switzerland), found that obesity rates for adult Europeans and Americans to be 17.1 percent and 33.1 percent, respectively. They also found that over half (53 percent) the latter, ex-or current smokers, versus 43 percent of the former, and that American adults were likelier to have chronic diseases, for examples, heart disease, cancer, diabetes, and chronic lung disease, correlated with obesity and smoking than Europeans were. There is no doubt that such findings would increasingly inform initiatives that healthcare strategies of firms in future would prescribe, such as those that would reduce the prevalence, the rates of all cases, and in particular, also their incidence, the rates of new cases, of conditions such as obesity and smoking, among their workers, without having to mandate them. No doubt, firms would likelier achieve that objective by fostering the voluntary collaboration of their workers in those initiatives, which for example, emphasizing empathy, would engender a sense of ownership that would in turn stimulate interest in such collaboration. Organization for Economic Cooperation and Development (OECD) data indicates that the U.S., spends more on healthcare than any country in Europe, in 2004, the country's per capita spending on healthcare, $6,102, nearly twice that of the Netherlands, Germany, and France9. The question then is why the U.S., seems to be getting less for its money than European countries are regarding healthcare. Are Americans less healthy? As one of the researchers noted, "It is possible that we spend more on health care because we are, indeed, less healthy. If the U.S. could bring its obesity rates more in line with Europe's, it could save $100 billion a year or more in health care costs." Indeed, they projected that the U.S could slash its per capita health spending by $1,195 to $1,750 per year, Americans age 50 and older diagnosed and treated at the lower European rates for 10 common chronic conditions namely, heart disease; high blood pressure; high cholesterol; stroke/cerebrovascular disease; diabetes; chronic lung diseases; asthma; arthritis; osteoporosis; and cancer9. According to the researchers, this could cut health spending by $100-$150 billion per year, or 12.7-18.7 percent off the total budget for personal health care spending for persons aged 50 and above. Could American firms, and indeed, those in other countries that are keen to achieve the DHDO learn something from these findings, regarding the need to focus on reducing the rates of certain conditions in particular, which is in fact doable, with attention to the tripartite disease prevention strategy mentioned earlier for example, and with an emphasis on initiatives unenforced? There could be a number of reasons for the differences in disease prevalence between Americans and Europeans, besides the former being unhealthier, for example, diagnosis and pretreatment of chronic diseases being more aggressive in the U.S., but this does not invalidate the need for firms to be proactive in their approaches to healthcare for their workers. In fact, this could only also be in the interests of the firms than otherwise. Furthermore, the researchers also noted that higher U.S. disease prevalence rates might vary by condition, Americans having more obesity-related disease markers, for examples, high blood pressure, suggesting that they are indeed, unhealthier than Europeans are, whereas having more cancer, twice as in Europe, likelier indicative of more intensive screening in the U.S. Both nonetheless suggest the need for firms, as we have here emphasized to undergo in-house, or perhaps outsourced, thorough process cycle and other analyses that would elucidate relevant health issues, and the most appropriate strategic approaches to them. That the researchers also observed that the differences in the prevalence of chronic diseases influenced the amount of medications and other treatments used for those diseases underscores this point. In fact, the lack of universal health coverage in the United States, regardless, Americans age 50 and older were likelier than European adults to receive drugs for six of nine diseases, including heart disease, diabetes, and asthma, an increase in treatment for chronic disease and medication use no doubt contributory to the country's soaring healthcare spending. This scenario would also doubtless ring true for many firms in the country, which further highlights the need for firms to pay sufficient attention to these issues, and seek the appropriate solutions to the problems in their peculiar contexts. Thus, the issue of mandating healthcare becomes not just one pertaining to governments imposing the mandate, but indeed, and perhaps more importantly, and in spite of such government mandates, what firms could do to achieve the DHDO without themselves falling prey, literally, to such tendencies as imposing mandates, health or any other, for that matter, on their workers.

The significance of healthcare for firms is already evident to the public given the publicity the negotiations between GM and UAW have attracted in recent times. What might not be so evident is that of employer-sponsored health insurance in the overall health system of any country, although it is doubtless that this would also become increasingly obvious in the years ahead. In countries such as the U.S., most Americans receive health insurance coverage via employer-sponsored plans, and many states actually want to expand access to employer-based insurance, some even mandating it. However, employers are expectedly concerned about increasing healthcare costs, not just on the 'wallet' but also in their global competitiveness. Premium contributions as a percentage of payroll is a focal point in the debate over the role of employers in health care reform, not surprisingly considering for example that although wages and salaries increased by 39 percent between 1996 and 2005, health insurance costs to employers increased 97 percent10. Furthermore, the percentage of total compensation paid as health insurance by firms that provide them increased from 6 to 8 percent from 1996 to 2005, the share of compensation paid as wages falling as health insurance costs rose, among these firms, costs relative to payroll also rose 34 percent during the same period 10. That unionized businesses, those that had most full-time workers, and those low-wage paid most premium contributions as a share of payroll, is also instructive, as is that despite the rise in health insurance costs being identical across businesses, low-wage firms had the most hikes. Indeed, in 2005, nearly 13 percent of low-wage businesses had premium contributions over 20 percent of payroll, versus almost 7 percent of high-wage firms. Thus, the least likely to keep offering coverage has most reasons not to, but also most reasons to have to given their role in the overall economy, not to mention that we need to encourage so to do, and not mandate out of so doing, if not even out of business. No doubt, a situation where employer premium contributions roughly doubled between 1996 and 2005, rising from $1,007 per worker to $1,979, would, in particular given the tendency to keep increasing, threaten firms, financially. This would be more in low-wage firms, where compensation has been relatively unchanged vis-à-vis high-wage firms, where it has increased significantly, part reason for higher increases in health insurance costs among the former. Thus, for employer-sponsored healthcare coverage to expand, the firms need to survive, to start with. These issues again, highlight the need for firms, large and small, to pursue the dual healthcare delivery objectives (DHDO) as a strategic imperative. The starting point being the determination to offer qualitative health services cost-effectively and efficiently would negate any tendency toward increased health spending that they could prevent, without compromising the quality of healthcare that their workers receive. Because healthcare becomes a strategic initiative, upon which the firm's survival predicates, achieving the DHDO would become standard objectives that firms would increasingly pursue, in so doing which would make evident, the importance of unforced involvement of the workers in making it possible to achieve the goals, and not any mandate to so do. There has not been much change in the U.S., over a ten-year period in the proportion of employers offering health benefits, actually just between 50 and 60 percent, doing so10. For the numbers to increase, conditions should prevail that ensures that these businesses thrive, and in fact, simply survive, which suggests that simply imposing a mandate on these firms without due considerations of the potential of such mandates to adversely affect businesses in the jurisdiction is anything but prudent. There is no doubt that such concerns would eventually feature prominently in decisions either by government or by the firms themselves to impose a healthcare mandate in one form or another, and indeed, discourage such moves. Not just firms need to worry about soaring health spending. A recent examination of changes in the affordability and covered benefits provided via California's individual and small group health insurance markets show ed that trends in premiums and covered benefits, relative to wages and income, indicate that affordability is a real and increasing concern for many insured individuals in the state11. According to the study, in these markets, where in fact, most currently uninsured Californians would obtain coverage, if they could pay for it, the costs of coverage and care is a significant percentage of income, especially for individual buyers. The health expenditures of such as a person in 2006 with median household income ($30,623) purchasing coverage in the individual market, 16 percent of income, in the small group market, 3.5 percent. The study also showed to pay lower monthly premiums one is responsible, in the individual market, for more of healthcare costs share, insurance coverage, 54.6 percent of a typical client's medical expenses, versus 83.3 percent in the small group market. Additionally, annual out-of-pocket medical expenses are high for persons with chronic conditions, in 2006, for one with diabetes, about $3,275 in the individual market, $1,101 in the small group market. These numbers indeed, suggest the increasing difficulties posed by the individual health insurance market, and the likelihood of an increasing shift toward the group market, which underscores that toward employer-sponsored healthcare coverage that we have here emphasized would happen sooner than later. Again, it brings to the fore the naivety of mandating healthcare coverage in one form or another, as opposed to promoting the pervasiveness of options in all aspects of healthcare, which would in turn foster creativity, improve healthcare delivery quality, and yet be affordable. The point here is that firms would have to embrace the need to conceptualize the idea of mandated healthcare and to view healthcare provision, as a working alliance between the firm and its workers, and which, as the other alliances between them, requires the collaboration of all involved. In other words, the symbiotic dyad that both create in matters of healthcare delivery, among others, should be the guiding principle of a partnership built on a shared sense of ownership of the processes and transactions involved in healthcare delivery, hence both responsible for their efficiency and cost-effectiveness. Thus, the question of mandating healthcare would be totally an anathema.

References:

1. Freudenheim, M. (2003, September 17). Many California Employers Face Health Care Mandate. Retrieved July 1, 2007 from,
http://query.nytimes.com/gst/fullpage.html?res=9D02E7DC143AF934A2575A

C0A9659C8B63&sec=health&spon=&pagewanted=print

2. Abelson R. In Health Care, Cost Isn't Proof of High Quality (2007, June 14). The New York Times. Retrieved July 01, 2007 from,

http://www.nytimes.com/2007/06/14/health/14insure.html?ei=5087%0A&em

=&en=b6885894907529c0&ex=1183435200&pagewanted=print

3. García-Lizana F, Sarría-Santamera A. New technologies for chronic disease management and control: a systematic review. J Telemed Telecare. 2007; 13(2):62- 8
4. Available at:

2007http://www.consumerwatchdog.org/resources/ltr_020807.pdf Accessed on July 01, 2007

5. Belluck, P. (2007, July 01.) Massachusetts Universal Care Plan Faces Hurdles. The New York Times. Retrieved on July 1, 2007 from

http://www.nytimes.com/2007/07/01/health/policy/01insure.html?ei=5087%

0A&em=&en=07885632e9e2b384&ex=1183435200&pagewanted=print

6. Available at:

http://www.freep.com/apps/pbcs.dll/article?AID=2007710050425 Accessed on October 6, 2007

7. Available at: http://archinte.ama-assn.org/ Accessed on October 6, 2007

8. Available at:

http://www.nytimes.com/2007/10/05/business/05conflict.html?_r=1&oref=slo gin Accessed on October 6, 2007

9. Available at:

http://content.healthaffairs.org/cgi/content/abstract/hlthaff.26.6.w678 Accessed on October 6, 2007

10. Eibner C, Kapur K, Marquis, MS. Snapshot: Employer Health Insurance Costs in the United States. California Healthcare Foundation. July 2007.

11. Snapshot Health Insurance: Can Californians Afford It? California Healthcare Foundation. June 2007

Healthcare Reform and Organizational Change

Interests in healthcare reform in the U.S have hardly been as intense as recently since the jettisoning in 1994 of President Bill Clinton's grand reform proposals. Fuelled by the ever-increasing health spending, the attrition of private insurance coverage, and the call from several quarters, including by corporate interests, organized labor, and other healthcare stakeholders for coverage expansion and to curtail health spending1, 2, 3, the clamour for more affordable healthcare coverage is ever louder. With the growth cuts in the two main public insurance initiatives, Medicare and Medicaid that the 2008 US budget proposes, would the corporate world be playing an even greater role in insurance coverage, and what would be the nature and extent of government involvement forthwith in this regard? These are indeed, questions applicable to many other countries, and given the real, or perceived threats of globalization, for example, should the private sector not be just as concerned as the public sector about the potential fallouts of ignoring health reforms? In the Organization for Economic Cooperation and Development's (OECD) 2007 annual Employment Outlook, it urged OECD governments to focus on improving labor regulations and social protection systems to help people adapt to job markets changes, rather than considering globalization as a threat. It also noted the chances that offshoring could have lessened workers' bargaining power, in particular low-skilled workers, and made jobs and salaries in developed countries more vulnerable4.

The increasing wage inequality since the early 1990s, also noted in the report in 18 of the 20 OECD countries where data was obtainable, including in the U.S, U.K, and Canada, the only exceptions, Ireland and Spain, could also have significant implications for healthcare coverage for workers and their families, even in those countries with publicly funded health systems. Indeed, the OECD recommendations for countries with high social security contributions such as Belgium, France and Sweden, include broadening the sources of financing public social protection, the organization arguing that social contributions being in the main wages-based, and a tax on labor, limit job creation. Furthermore, with wages share in national income declining, a reduction of the role of social contributions is apt, as is tax bases broadening, for examples, income taxes and/or VAT, for social protection funding4. Do these recommendations have any bearings on the contention by some of the need for increasing private sector involvement in healthcare delivery, and what could this mean for coverage expansion, or otherwise? In other words, would individuals in such countries rather not have to pay more taxes, and prefer having more latitude to deal with their health matters? On the other hand, the U.S for example, depends on 'unforced', employer-sponsored health insurance to fund healthcare coverage for workers and their dependents, 68.2% of all workers in 2005, covered by private insurance, 59.5%, employer-sponsored, just 27.5%, of all insured in the country government-sponsored5. It is thus, understandable, the 'new' push for universal coverage in the country, given private insurance being increasingly less affordable, fewer businesses offering it, even increasingly fewer workers with such coverage. 15.9% of the US population, 46.6 million individuals, did not have health insurance coverage in 2005, about 70%, adults, with incomes below 200% of the federal poverty level, in 2007, $20,650 for a family of four5. What is less clear is the role that businesses would play in this regard, and for that matter, what this role would imply for organizational change, and what form this would take. It is also uncertain if individuals, including workers in the U.S would rather pay more taxes rather than have more private sector involvement in healthcare coverage. Another OECD document, Regions at a Glance 20075, noted that a region's and indeed, a country's growth prospects hinge in part on its ability to generate and use innovation, which in turn depends on its labor force's skills levels, in particular in contemporary knowledge-based economies. That for example, regional variations in educational levels are substantial among OECD countries, is instructive. In France, Australia, the U.K, and Canada differences in tertiary educational accomplishments between the best and worst-performing regions are over 30 percentage points5, and generally, urban regions perform better than intermediate, or rural ones, 57% of the OECD adult population that have a tertiary education resident in urban regions. What organizational changes would businesses in urban and rural regions need to make in playing a role in this regard for the economy to thrive? This is more so given also that in about half the countries surveyed, except Austria, Denmark, Greece and Spain, males living in rural regions likelier died prematurely, in part because of the higher fatal traffic accidents rates on country roads. Could such changes also be relevant for the national and regional variations also observed in smoking and obesity rates, for example, and that among females, those living in urban areas were at higher risk, particularly in Austria, Denmark, Japan and Poland? In other words, would the changes include attention to a blend of education and health related issues, rather than simply one or the other, and would considerations of these issues, among others, include for all those for whom businesses sponsor health insurance and other benefits, and indeed, their dependants? These questions highlight the contention of some, for example, Michigan University's Economic Research Initiative on the Uninsured, Helen Levy, and David Meltzer of the University of Chicago that there is no evidence that expanding coverage is cost-effective in improving health, and that other means exist that could procure more health for the funds used 6. Indeed, other researchers have noted that neither would expanding coverage increase overall longevity, healthcare quality, nor would it eradicate health disparities across races and socio-economic groups, or stop free-riders6. They also underscore the significance of an all-inclusive approach to corporate healthcare reform strategies, given first though, an appreciation by businesses of the need for participating in such reforms, and the conceptualization of the reforms at the corporate level as integral to those proposed and implemented in the wider society. There is for example in the US, potent bipartisan support, which the need for Congress to reauthorize the State Children's Health Insurance Program (SCHIP) underpins, for legislation aimed at expanding coverage focusing on children in 2007, in particular given that the legal mandate for SCHIP expires on September 30, 2007, despite the Presidential veto. Would it therefore not be counterintuitive for businesses to discountenance such moves, in formulating their strategies for healthcare coverage for their workers and their families, in not just the curative but also the preventive domains for examples? Furthermore, with mobility an essential aspect of globalization for example, would more countries be adopting Austria and Denmark's "flexicurity" approach, in the former, workers with personal savings accounts, not the customary severance pay schemes, that move with them with job changes, able to withdraw from it, if they lost their job, or save up towards a future pension4. Should employers also not consider compensating job losers via employment-friendly, social protection systems? Indeed, OECD suggests this is achievable by providing adequate benefits hand-in-hand with "activation" policies that augment re-employment prospects, policies, which based on what transpired in Nordic countries and Australia, well designed, could significantly enhance laid-off workers' re-employment prospects, allaying globalization concerns4. The point here is that the stakes are increasing regarding issues such as health, and indeed, social protection systems, for businesses and their workers alike, and would equally increasingly demand a comprehensive conceptualization of the various issues involved, for which strategic formulations would result in potentially far-reaching organizational changes. In other words, businesses would need to give serious considerations not just to their healthcare strategies, but also the interplay of these strategies with relevant developments in other domains, within and outside their businesses with the potential not jus to affect their healthcare strategies, but their businesses in general. This would require the adoption of the appropriate mind set not just at the executive decision making level, but across the enterprise, the initiation of a new culture resultant, compatible with the recognition of the importance for the survival, let alone progress of the business, upon which both employers and employees depend for their livelihood, not to mention stockholders' interests. In so doing, businesses would be acquiescing to healthcare being central to the success of their operations, and indeed, in the bigger picture, literally, that of the economy of the jurisdictions in which they operate too. This places the onus on these businesses to spearhead the appropriate initiatives to ensure that their workers receive qualitative health services, affordably, and to create the enabling atmosphere for the workers to buy-in into these initiatives, and in general, the new culture that the firm is attempting for all in it to imbibe. This situation would involve comprehensive structural and functional organizational changes. As the foregoing implies, to accomplish these changes would require the collaboration of all, and would be anything but a top-down, hierarchical, compensation-rooted, instructional approach, and would need appropriate expertise to manage depending upon the nature and extent of the imminent changes.

No doubt, the objectives of businesses would be to ensure that the transition from the old to the new culture proceeds smoothly, and that the firm and its workers both achieve their respective goals, which essentially coincide with regard to healthcare provision. In other words, both want cost-effective and efficient qualitative health services provision, the quintessential dual healthcare delivery objectives (DHDO), which would require for example, changes in behaviour of individuals such as embracing a healthy lifestyle. It would also require some changes in the firm, for example, paying more attention to health issues, particularly new research studies and their applications to their workers and organizations, or even building an onsite gym, designing new work processes, investing in new technologies, or organizing health education workshops on diet, and stress, for instance, for its staff. There are of course a number of theories of individual change management. They include those of Lewin7 and Elizabeth Kubler-Ross8, and of Richard Beckhard/ David Gleicher's Gleicher's Formula 9and the ADKAR model10 with its five building blocks namely; Awareness, of the need for change; Desire, to support and participate in it; Knowledge, of the way to change; Ability, to practice new skills and behaviours and; Reinforcement, to maintain the change. There are also a number of ideas of organizational change, and of mechanisms and tools for achieving it, some structured, others semi-structured, and yet others, informal approaches. David Cooperrider's Appreciative Inquiry (AI) 11, for example is an organizational development process that emphasizes collaboration in the change process11. Its 4-stage process namely: discover, the discovery of effective organizational processes; dream, figuring those that would; design, with an emphasis on those processes and; destiny/deliver, the execution of planned design, are increasingly employed by businesses. Its focus on implementing change to improve the organization rather than being stuck with outmoded processes is resonant with the position we here stress regarding the desirability, and indeed, imperativeness of change. Many of these ideas and theories have roots in human psychology, the continuing evolution in knowledge of which underscores not only the point about the need for firms to be conversant with developments in their domains and others, in relation to health, but why our focus here would not be to dig deep into these theories and ideas. Rather, we would examine the larger picture of the interplay of the health reform/organizational change dyad, the latter component conceptualized generically, as integrative of the elements involved with the drivers and management of change at the individual and organizational levels. Thus, we would focus more on what businesses ought to know about health reform and developments in the health and related sectors that could necessitate a variety of changes in their organizations. In other words, to recognize, firstly, that change is imperative, and in fact desirable, given that in implementing the appropriate responses to observed developments and trends in their macro-and micro-environments, they would likely be setting their organizations up for success rather than failure in an increasingly competitive global business climate. The details of how these changes would affect their workers, processes, and technologies, and indeed, their relations with say, their suppliers, are also crucial to know, which they would need in some instances, a change management expert to assist in deciphering and managing. As noted earlier, suffice to reiterate here the importance of collaboration among all concerned for the smooth transitioning in the change process, and its overall success eventually, which process would require effective supervision and monitoring, and the implementation of required modifications to achieve this success. Regardless of the organizational configurations therefore, its essential humanity is what drives the success of its healthcare reform initiatives, its tendency to earn the trust of its workers in recognizing the proposed changes as being not just in the organization's interests, but also in those of the workers. This explains the difference at least in part between individuals that recognize the need for adopting a healthy lifestyle and those that not only do so, but also actually adopt the necessary changes that such a lifestyle warrants. In other words, organizations would increasingly realize that the organizational changes required for the achievement of the dual healthcare delivery objectives for example would hardly materialize if at all, the organization sticking with the old mentality of enforcing compliance via compensation, for example. Workers in future, and in an increasingly globalized economy, and 'material' world, in which labor is ever more mobile, and workers have multiple income streams would be hard-pressed to volunteer their loyalty to any firm, in particular based simply on compensation-based enforcement of company regulations. Yet, these firms would need to continue to strive to achieve their stated goals, no matter how temporary their workforce becomes. This would necessitate the sort of change in mindset that we mentioned earlier that would permeate strategic orientation in health and indeed, other matters. The nature of the approaches adopted by firms would need to match the reality of their particular vision and the prospects and challenges of achieving it in their particular jurisdictions on the one hand, and within the context of the global economy, on the other. Underlying the organizational change that they would undergo however, would have to be a strong emphasis on creating an environment in which trust between workers and employers is possible, a requirement for workers to develop a sense of ownership in the proposed healthcare initiatives impelled by change.

Organizations would therefore, need to detect developments/changes in their internal and external environment on the one hand, and seek the trust, hence collaboration of their workers in implementing the necessary changes in their processes, to ensure the sustainability of their operations that the continuing and perhaps even enhanced productivity that a healthy and vibrant workforce assures. Even with their best efforts, firms would also need to deal with resistance to change, which might be due to an innate fear of change due to threats to the status quo, conservatism intrinsic in humans possibly linked to fear of the unknown. Kotter and Schlesinger12, 13, 14, also noted four reasons why some people resist change namely: parochial self-interest; misunderstanding; low change tolerance; and differences of opinions on the need for and approach to change, and suggested that education; participation and involvement; facilitation and support; negotiation and agreement; manipulation and co-option; and explicit/implicit coercion as ways by means to address resistance to change. There are indeed, approaches to managing resistance to change that firms would devise based on their peculiar contexts, although as we have here noted, regardless of time constraints, as Kotter and Schlesinger noted its use might be appropriate when pressed for time, we do not consider that coercion would achieve the desired results for the reasons earlier mentioned. Furthermore, firms could reduce the chances of such resistance developing by involving the workers and their representatives in the proposed initiatives right from conceptualization through its entire life cycle. In other words, it might not be enough for a firm, recognizing the need for its workers to maintain healthy weights to build a gym onsite without input from the workers on whether they would prefer for example, financial assistance from their employers to purchase their individual treadmills, for example. It is possible that it would be cheaper for the firm to contribute say 25% of the costs of the treadmill than build the onsite gym, after all to start with, not to mention the likelier prospects of realizing the stated goals as workers, with part of the cost coming from their pockets, likely exercise on the treadmill. In fact, the treadmill would be there for their family members to use as well, not just keeping workers and their families healthy, but also in fact, potentially saving the firm, the workers, healthcare costs, both able to achieve the DHDO. It is conceivable that enforcing the use of the gym might make some but unlikely all workers use it, not to mention the disharmony that would ensue, which could compromise loyalty, and indeed, productivity. Thus, firms would need to implement their own local health reforms in a manner of speaking to apply the results of research studies to ensuring the well-being of their workers. The reasons for the firm promoting the adoption of a healthy life style should be paramount in the communication between the establishment and the workers. In other words, businesses would increasingly have to be proactive in letting its workers know why it is embarking on any health reform initiative, including preparing relevant memos containing a digest of the research and other data and information that prompted the initiative. We see therefore that that organizations would need a reorientation, which would make such communications routine, what we referred to as the functional change that they would need to undergo as part of the overall organizational change in mindset required for survival, let alone, progress in an ever-more competitive business milieu. Thus, this functional change would complement any structural change, for example in the organizational structure, required to make the necessary transitions that change itself impels. Indeed, it would be necessary for firms to accept the inevitability of change and the need to make the necessary adjustments to accommodate them, particularly driven by what many would deem the feverish pace of progress in medicine, itself in association of that in technology.

To keep abreast of developments in Medicine therefore, and indeed, in other domains relevant to healthcare delivery, for examples, the insurance and pharmaceutical industries, in any bid to ensure that they make the necessary organizational adjustments to address the issues consequent upon the change successfully, we would likely see more firms developing healthcare strategies with more vigour. As noted earlier, education is likely going to a crucial aspect of these strategies, as workers would need current and reliable health information, in addition to data and information on healthcare providers. They would also need information on pricing of health services, among others for them to make rational decisions on service utilization, which they would prefer to do increasingly as firms are better able to establish the trust that engender such commitments. In addition, it would be easier for workers to appreciate the need for prudence that their employers also stress, approaching the matter from the perspective of someone who also has a stake in the survival of the firm, in addition to not emptying their individual pockets paying for health services that they do not need. It is evident therefore that the adoption of a positive stand by firms toward healthcare strategies would be beneficial to the firms and their workers in the long term, at least. Thus, one of the key healthcare initiatives that firms would engage in would be rectifying the pervasive information asymmetry in the health sector, its long history, and roots in the paternalism equally pervasive among healthcare professionals notwithstanding. This is not to say that doctors might still not know more about health conditions, and that workers would still not rely on and obtain a significant amount of the health information that they need from doctors. On the contrary, and as even doctors, themselves increasingly recognize, there is such an information glut on medical subjects out there that no one, doctors or not, could claim to have a monopoly of knowledge on medical issues these days. Besides, there are sources, for example, on the Internet, dedicated to providing health information to individuals in ways in which they could assimilate this information, perhaps even better than how their doctors and other healthcare professionals present it. Depending on the resources available to a firm therefore, we would likely start to see firms collaborating with some of these Internet health information providers to source health information for their workers, perhaps via the organization's intranet. This might in fact be one way for firms that prohibit their workers to surf the Internet during working hours to have limited access to the Internet, or intranet as the case may be perhaps even at stipulated times, to prevent such access, carried out in excess, compromising productivity. Alternatively, firms might provide their workers with a password to access web sites at home funded by the firm, to enable the workers access such health information as would facilitate rational decision making on health issues by the workers. We would also likely see the increasing use of the Internet, and in fact other healthcare information and communications technologies (healthcare ICT) by firms, for other healthcare delivery purposes for their workers. For examples, firms might again collaborate with technology solutions providers to enable their workers utilize healthcare ICT for the management of chronic diseases, such as diabetes, heart diseases, and asthma. Several studies attest to the effectiveness of these technologies in managing chronic diseases[15, 16]. A recent systematic review of studies for example showed that ICTs utilized in the detection and follow up of cardiovascular diseases provided improved clinical outcomes, and reduced mortality and health services use. It also showed that systems used for improving education and social supports were effective[15]. The findings of another study, on Interactive Health Communication Applications (IHCAs), computer-based, typically web-based, information packages for patients that combine health information with at least one of social support, decision support, or behaviour change support, aimed at benefits in health care and their effects on health for people with chronic disease are instructive[16]. The authors found that IHCAs seem to have mostly 'positive effects on users, in that users tend to become more knowledgeable, feel better socially supported, and may have improved behavioural and clinical outcomes compared to non-users.' They recommended 'more high quality studies with large sample sizes to confirm these preliminary findings, to determine the best type and best way to deliver IHCAs, and to establish how IHCAs have their effects for different groups of people with chronic illness,' the outcomes of which studies firms should also be keen to know. Given the increasing influence of these technologies on medical practice at all levels, including in the prevention and treatment of diseases, it is unlikely that firms would be able to ignore developments in technological progress as well, as they would not in medical progress. In fact, they would need to integrate such knowledge ever more in their healthcare strategies, as these technologies have the potential to facilitate the achievement by these firms of the dual healthcare delivery objectives mentioned earlier. The applications of these technologies might mean embarking on structural organizational changes in the physical sense, for examples, investing in additional broadband capacities, or in security solutions, to secure the privacy of the health information of their workers to which they have access. This issue of privacy would loom large increasingly over firms' healthcare strategies in particular, further underscoring the need for firms to adopt a benign approach that emphasizes trust building between workers and their employees to ensure their collaboration in initiatives that might require information gathering for the successful implementation of particular elements of the firms' healthcare strategies. For instance, a firm might want to encourage its workers to use personal health records (PHRs), which would make critical health information available to authorized healthcare personnel, say the in-house company doctor that treats minor ailments onsite, or that is involved in the company's preventive cardiology program, or even physiotherapy program. There might be the need for the company to invest in technologies that would enable access to such information without compromising its security, or making it vulnerable to hackers and identity thieves on the Internet/Intranet. Given the sensitivity of private health information, success in the use of healthcare ICT by firms to achieve their healthcare strategy objectives would depend mainly on how much the firms could allay the anxieties of their workers regarding such use. Still on these technologies, firms would likely increasingly exploit their potential to improve the efficiencies of healthcare delivery to their workers predicated on a variety of healthcare delivery dimensions, which would involve them changing how the interface with for examples health plans, and healthcare providers. Besides, the likely increasing interests of firms in the population health approach to healthcare delivery, specifically in the utilization of healthcare ICT in the primary, secondary, and tertiary prevention of diseases, some of which we have mentioned above, they would be keen to see how these technologies help them achieve the DHDO in other ways. One such way is in ensuring accountability on the parts of the other players in the healthcare delivery dynamics, such as insurers, doctors, and pharmacies, not only in seeking transparencies in pricing but also in being able to compare prices, and in ensuring that professionals have proper licensing and are in good standing for examples in their professions. The deployment of the appropriate technologies that would facilitate the achievement of these goals would require both functional and structural organizational changes the nature and extent of which vary with the size of the firm, its wherewithal financial, and otherwise, and its overall strategic objectives.

Considering the potential for transactions in the service industry to be quite expensive, not least in healthcare delivery, with its variety of transactions, and professionals involve therein, the close monitoring of these transactions with a view to making them more efficient, hence more cost-effective, would increasingly gain the attention of firms. It would also necessitate these firms investing in the relevant technologies. Consider a recent article, anticipating the debate in the U.S House on health legislation, the "CHAMP Act", developed by the chairs of the House Energy and Commerce and the House Ways and Means Committees to reauthorize and expand the State Children's Health Insurance Program (SCHIP), and curtail excessive payments made to private insurance plans under the Medicare Advantage program 17. CHAMP Act means Children's Health and Medicare Protection Act of 2007 (H.R. 3162, as introduced). The author noted that private plans were firstly introduced into the Medicare program to cut costs. He further noted that however, the Medicare Payment Advisory Commission (MedPAC), Congress' expert advisory body on Medicare payment policy, and the

Congressional Budget Office have noted that 'private plans are paid 12 percent more, on average, than it would cost traditional Medicare to cover the same beneficiaries17. The author added that as a correctional measure, MedPAC has recommended over the years that Congress set payments to private plans at the same levels, as it would cost to serve comparable beneficiaries under the traditional Medicare program, a recommendation approved by many Medicare beneficiary advocacy groups. These groups included the AARP, the American Medical Association, the National Committee to Preserve Social Security and Medicare. The CHAMP Act would in effect adopt the MedPAC recommendation, which according to preliminary Congressional Budget Office estimates, in addition to other House provisions aimed at curtailing overpayments to private plans would result in savings of $50.2 billion over the next five years17. No doubt, healthcare ICT would play a crucial role in the health reforms on which firms would ever more of necessity engage in, as these technologies become more an integral part of healthcare delivery, if not indeed, essential to its continuing survival. This is more so, as with businesses, governments around the world cannot afford to let their healthcare budgets keep escalating, if indeed, they would be able to continue to manage them, in the first place, which increasingly seems unlikely, for those costs reasons, and for the fact the employer-sponsored health insurance would become predominant with time. This highlights the need and indeed, away from which firms would not be able to shy, literally, for these firms to be more attuned to the role that they would increasingly play in healthcare delivery not only to their workers, but in the health systems in their respective jurisdictions in general in the years ahead.

We have conceptualized health reform here in its generic sense, as initiatives necessary in view of changes in medicine, technology, and other domains, and in the micro-and macro-environments of firms that would influence their healthcare strategies, and the initiatives emanating thereof. We have used the term organizational change in an equally generic sense. This reflects the broad-based approach to conceptualizing these issues that firms would also need to adopt to facilitate attention to the various dimensions of these issues necessary to address them successfully. Thus, firms would need to discard the hierarchical organizational mindset to be successful in devising not just the appropriate healthcare strategies but also in ensuring their effective implementation. They would need for, to attune to developments such as Web 2.0 to capitalize on the benefits of social networking as an option in the dissemination of health information among their workers for example. They should be ready to utilize whatever avenues they deem appropriate for communicating with their workers, some of which might reflect the appreciation of the firms of the developments in domains outside of theirs but nonetheless invaluable portals for information dissemination to their workers based, for example on preference characteristic of the particular jurisdiction in which the firm operates. Thus, firms would need to be flexible in their approaches to healthcare strategies, and be agile in modifying their organizations to meet the challenges posed by change. Regardless of the specific focus of these firms, they would all still have to address two principal generic issues, which are to provide qualitative health services to their workers, and to do so, cost-effectively and efficiently. Thus, they would all need to try to achieve the dual healthcare delivery objectives mentioned above. In other words, their healthcare strategies would generically aim to achieve these dual goals. The differences would predicate on such factors as demographics, disease prevalence, the availability or otherwise of technology and other infrastructures and institutions, the health financing model in their operational jurisdictions, and the regulations therein, among others. These factors would interplay with some, generic factors, for example, progress in medicine and technology, some of which developments firms would need to adapt to suit their particular needs. Thus, firms would have to factor into their healthcare strategies, the age distribution of their workers, and the differential prevalence of diseases related to age, and other factors such as heredity, race, and gender in their approaches to developing the relevant initiatives, which would directly, or otherwise, influence the operations of their organizations. These factors for example might influence the nature, type, and rate of medical examinations that the firm's medical department if it had any, or medical doctor, would recommend that certain workers have annually or at some specified intervals. As earlier noted, this of course implies no compulsion, but suggestions and encouragement in the manner earlier discussed, something that would likely yield the desired results the appropriate approaches adopted, flexibly incorporating cutting-edge knowledge in change management for example, perhaps, involving experts in consultation on such issues the firm's finances permitting. The point here is that firms would need to increasingly become objective in their approaches to realizing their healthcare delivery goals, and ensure that such goals coincide at least in principle with those of their workers to ensure the harmony, and commitment that is the underlying strand in their healthcare strategy. In other words, this commitment is the result of their healthcare strategy that would ensure enhanced productivity, which a healthy workforce enables to begin with. Thus, the goals of firms would not simply be to ensure that they have a healthy workforce, but that this workforce is productive, and committed to the progress of the firm. This brings to the fore the emphasis we have placed on securing the trust of workers and engendering a sense of ownership of the firm in them right from the onset being crucial to the success of a company's healthcare strategy, and the benefits it expects the strategy to bestow. It also underscores the possible need for organization changes that the realization of this trust and commitment would warrant as could the changes the healthcare initiatives arising thereof could. In all, the successful firm in future would need to pay attention to the issues we have here and more to ensure that it exploits the potential in its workforce to enhance its chances of becoming and remain viable in an increasingly highly competitive global economy. Health is no longer what firms could take for granted and indeed, ignore, as employer-sponsored health insurance takes center stage literally in the health system of countries, ever more in the years to come.

References:

1. Unprecedented alliance of health care leaders announces historic agreement to help reduce the numbers of America's uninsured. News release from the Health Coverage Coalition for the Uninsured. (Accessed July 10, 2007, at http://www.coalitionfortheuninsured.org.)

2. We believe every American should have access to affordable health care coverage: a vision for reform. Washington, DC: America's Health Insurance Plans. (Accessed July 10, 2007, at http://www.ahipbelieves.com/vision-for-reform.html.)

3. FAH unveils "Health Coverage Passport" to insure all Americans. News release from the Federation of American Hospitals, Washington, DC.

4. Accessed July 10, 2007, at

http://www.oecd.org/document/12/0,3343,en_2649_201185_38792716_1_1_1_1,

00.html

5. DeNavas-Walt C, Proctor BD, Lee CH. Income, poverty, and health insurance coverage in the United States: 2005. Washington, DC: Census Bureau, 2006.

6. Accessed July 10, 2007, at

http://www.cato.org/pub_display.php?pub_id=8199

7. Lewin, K. (1951). Field Theory in Social Science. New York: Harper and Row.

8. Kubler-Ross, E. 1970. On Death and Dying, Macmillan Company, England.

9. Beckhard, R. 1969. Organization Development: Strategies and Models, Addison- Wesley, Reading, MA.

10. Hiatt, J. 2006. ADKAR: A Model for Change in Business, Government and the Community, Learning Center Publications, Loveland, CO

11. Kinni T, "The Art of Appreciative Inquiry", The Harvard Business School Working Knowledge for Business Leaders Newsletter, September 22, 2003.

12. Kotter, J. P., Schlesinger P.F. Organization: text, cases, and readings on the management of organizational design and change. 3rd ed. Homewood, IL: Irwin, 1992.

13. Kotter, J. P., Schlesinger L.A, Sathe, V. Organization: Text, Cases, and Readings on the Management of Organization Design and Change. 2nd ed. Homewood, Ill.: Richard D. Irwin, 1986.

14. Schlesinger, P. F., Schlesinger, L.A., Sathe, V., Kotter, J.P. Organization: Text, Cases, and Readings on the Management of Organization Design and Change. 3rd ed. Homewood, Ill.: Richard D. Irwin Inc., 1992.

15. García-Lizana F, Sarría-Santamera A. New technologies for chronic disease management and control: a systematic review. J Telemed Telecare. 2007; 13(2):62- 8

16. Murray E, Burns J, See TS, Lai R, Nazareth I. Interactive Health Communication Applications for people with chronic disease. Cochrane Database Syst. Rev. 2005 Oct 19 ;(4):CD004274

17. Available at:

http://pdftohtml.markoer.org/pdf2html.php?url=http%3A%2F%2Fwww.cbpp.org%2F7-31-07health4.pdf&images=yes Accessed on October 7, 2007

Prospects and Challenges of Employer-Based Health Insurance

Some health systems such as that of the U.S. depend substantially on employers to provide health insurance coverage to their workers, nearly 175 million Americans currently so provided for an essential aspect of the employees' total remuneration package, although nearly 47 million other Americans, 16% of the population, did not have health insurance in 20051. However, mounting health care costs continue to pose major challenges to employer-sponsored health insurance. Escalating costs are also at least in part responsible for about 47 million Americans lacking any health insurance. Thomas A. Scully, Administrator, Centers for Medicare and Medicaid Services (CMS) in a testimony on strengthening and improving Medicare given on Friday, June 06, 2003 before the Senate Finance Committee, noted that Medicare is a binding commitment to society's most vulnerable citizens, which obligation it should keep 2. Many would argue that employers ought to consider the provision of health benefits to their workers as also a commitment. With the participation of businesses in healthcare provision increasingly determined by statute that make such participation mandatory, what challenges might this pose to the ability of these businesses to negotiate rates to providers based on such indices as differential price of services and products, their volume, and in particular, also their quality? Could these challenges further aggravate costs and compromise profitability, even survival for these firms? No doubt, the variables involved in the appropriate determination of such rates would depend mainly on local market conditions, which raises the question of the extent to which the federal or any government should participate in making such local market-level differentiations. Besides this being a key Medicare reform consideration it is one that has major significance for the involvement of employers in healthcare provision given the increasing interests in the country in universal healthcare, and in some states, in mandating it. Yet, employers would also need to track developments in the private healthcare marketplace, including their local nuances. That the healthcare consumer having more options and providers enhancing offerings could weigh heavily on the outcomes of healthcare delivery, in not just efficiency and cost-effectiveness terms, but also regarding its overall quality and in meeting the expectations in fact, of enrolees, purchasers, and providers alike, for example, is instructive. Yet, so is that businesses in addressing their workers' healthcare needs would recognize increasingly the need to attend to the value proposition of providers, in making choices, as they would the possible negation of the potential for improved healthcare delivery outcomes that constraints on ensuring the optimization of the benefits accruable from the options implied in such attention, might mean. The overall effect of this state of affairs would be adverse on workers and their employers, with healthcare costs further driven upwards. There is no gainsaying not aggravating the problems that employer-sponsored health insurance on which, as in the US, many depend face. In fact, the need to tackle them successfully is urgent, given the imperfections of the country's health system, and their ramifications for society and the country's economy, concerns that hold in many other countries, developed or otherwise. Indeed, these countries would increasingly need to consider the benefits of competition and free-market operations in health services provision, even with universal coverage the overriding goal. A situation for example wherein doctors, hospitals, and providers receive federally determined flat rates for services provided, would unlikely inspire excellence, which requires a more than average dose of positive attitude and zeal. Hence, even with universal coverage, performance-based incentives, for example, among others, would likely boost service quality, hence reduce overall healthcare costs, hence spending. These issues are elements of contemporary healthcare delivery we cannot afford to ignore. In other words, as desirable and important as coverage is, it is not, in itself, the panacea for the ills of any country's health system, if there was any to begin with. On the other hand, that the pursuit of the dual healthcare delivery objectives (DHDO), the provision of qualitative, accessible and affordable health services to all, cost-effectively, and efficiently, and indeed, curtailing soaring health spending, should be pervasive, is in keeping with the appropriate outlook to these ills. This would make the choice, for example, of health plan, say in the US between Preferred Provider Organizations (PPOs), and Fee-For-Service plans (FFS), more rational. Such choices for instance might predicate on the healthcare consumer's expectations of care, the provider's value proposition, including for example, the provision of preventive health services, or the utilization of healthcare information and communication technologies (healthcare ICT) to enhance service delivery and reduce costs, issues of which employers would increasingly be cognizant. The number of Americans that employer-sponsored health insurance covered fell from 70.4% in 1999 to 68.2% in 2002, mostly due to economic downturn starting 2000 and higher health insurance costs[3], low-income families affected the most, which underscores the potential benefits of the Medicaid expansion program in Oregon, The Oregon Health Plan (OHP), Oregon's Section 1115 Medicaid waiver program [4]. However, it also does, some of the issues involved in such expansion, in this case to all residents living below the poverty line. Enrolling 64 percent of the potentially eligible population in 1996[5], it the program peaked in its second year, with more than 134,000 eligibles, declining to just over 81,000 by January 1999 the end of its fifth year[4]. That even though the decline pertained mostly to new families and adults/couples, it was more marked, between July 1997 and July 1998, among new families is instructive, in part, because the States Children Health Insurance Program (SCHIP) implemented in the state moved children out of the 'new families' category. However, and perhaps equally importantly, the Medicaid expansion program also declined following the imposition of a premium requirement, economic upturn, and a number of other changes in eligibility requirements[4]. Furthermore, it did not eliminate Oregon's uninsured problem, as despite the rate falling to 17% in 1996, an estimated 23% of Oregonians living below poverty still lacked health insurance in 1998[6]. The Oregon program did not crowd-out private insurance, but it did not show either that employer-sponsored health insurance coverage is not susceptible to economic setbacks, despite the potential for such public program expansions to absorb the numbers of the otherwise uninsured. In fact, it showed the potential for cost-sharing, which many firms would prefer than outright health insurance sponsorship for their workers, to diminish enrolment in a health plan, or encourage care-shunning, both with likely adverse effects on health, and potentially on productivity. Furthermore, it is arguable that the costs implications of expansion in public coverage, Medicaid expenditures, for instance, increasing from $202 billion in 2000 to $257 billion in 2002, due partly to more children and non-disabled adults enrolled, also given the resultant budget pressures at state and federal levels, if unchecked, or aggravated, would offset[7] the decline in employer-sponsored coverage, eventually. This is more considering employers, particularly the small businesses, which bear a significant portion of the burden of employer sponsored coverage, have financial pressures of their own, including those due to rising health insurance premiums. With many of the firms offering coverage requesting higher cost-sharing from employees resulting in many employees unable to afford it opting out of such coverage, expansion in public coverage cost-intensive, and unlikely sustainable ad infinitum, healthcare stakeholders face an urgent pressure for answers to this quagmire. This again, brings to the fore, the need to recognize and implement the underlying principles of the DHDO, for example, among others, generic and specific, to address successfully, the challenges that contemporary healthcare delivery poses. The starting point, including for businesses is to appreciate in full, the fundamental basis of the commitment to healthcare provision mentioned earlier, and to acknowledge it, which would make the prospects of such commitment for the realization of their strategic objectives clear, including survivability, let alone profitability. Also clear, would be the constraints in realizing them, in the US for example, the number of uninsured up by 1.3 million in 2004/ 05, by about7 million since 20001, in 2005, mostly working age adults, 18.5% of those 18 to 64 years, lacking health coverage in 2004, 20.5% in 20051 when about a million permanent employees lost their health coverage. That in the country in 2005, almost 15% of employees lacked employer-sponsored health insurance, on their own or courtesy a family member8, and that about 30% of US companies did not provide healthcare coverage in 20059, has implications for not just the affected individuals, but for the country's economy overall, would also register markedly in our 'actionable' lists. In other words, there are indeed, solutions to the healthcare delivery problems, in not just the US, but also in other countries, if only the will to ferret out these solutions from their cryptic depths and implement them is not lacking. A major challenge that businesses in these countries would increasingly confront is whether to wager in the conundrum real or imagined that they would otherwise situate. Yet, overcoming this challenge does not necessarily have to be a chore. In fact, following the appreciation in full of the fundamental basis of the commitment to healthcare coverage to the workers that they should embrace is another to principles emanating thereof crucial to this commitment materializing. In other words, rather than as is the case with firms, particularly the smaller firms, not offering health coverage due to soaring costs of health insurance premiums, firms embrace the need to provide their workers with health insurance coverage as sine qua non to their, the firms', very survival.

Thus, firms would benefit from employer-sponsored health insurance in many ways. It is likely that they would increasingly realize this and devise appropriate ways to ensure the provision of health services for their workers rather than shy away from it, literally. How long it would take this to happen on a large scale and in many countries is conjectural, but it would no doubt happen. In fact, the smarter firms would sooner appreciate the competitive edge derivable from developing a healthcare strategy and a framework from which to approach the issues pertaining to health services provision for their workers that would assure them such advantage. Besides the prospects of a healthy workforce that would enhance a firm's productivity, the cultivation of the appropriate corporate culture whose expression would buoy the firm's strategic objectives in health services provision, but also permeate other aspects of life in the firm. For example, it would foster trust and a sense of ownership from which would spring loyalty, and commitment to the ideals of the firm, to which ascribing a price would no doubt be difficult. Besides promoting the health of its workers, such a firm would also be doing so directly or otherwise for their families, the psychological and physical well-being resultant, likely to rub off, literally, on their family members, who would likely imbibe the positive attitude that has patently made such a remarkable difference to the health of the index person, the worker. The domino effect of this scenario on their friends, their neighbours, and to society in general is not difficult to conceptualize. To underscore this point, when one hears that obesity is infectious, the first thing that would come to mind in all likelihood would be that some bug might be responsible for obesity. Indeed, recent research evidence suggests that a virus might be associated with obesity, an idea that gained currency after in 2005, the Pennington Biomedical Research Centre in Louisiana formed the first department of viruses and obesity in the U.S., the term, 'infectobesity' also coined Dr. Nikhil Dhurandhar, its head10. While Dhurandhar's focus is on adenoviruses, other researchers including microbiologists at Washington

University in St. Louis more interested in the role of microbes in our intestines in obesity. Yet, it is in the role of social factors in obesity that bears immediate significance for our discussion at this point. With millions of individuals in both developed and developing countries either overweight or obese, many of these persons workers, roughly a third of Americans for example obese, there should doubtless be cause for concern. Indeed, the U.S., Department of Health and Human Services indicated that obesity may be responsible for 300,000 deaths annually, the second commonest preventable cause of death, cigarette smoking, not to mention its association with a number of different diseases such as hypertension, diabetes, heart disease, sleep apnea, gallbladder disease, even cancers and osteoarthritis. According to the department on its Web site, "Individuals, who are obese, have a 50 to 100 percent increased risk of premature death from all causes, compared to individuals with a healthy weight." 10 Is it not striking therefore that our family and friends could give us obesity? No doubt, obesity runs in families, hence has a genetic component too. A recent study noted that the risk of obesity rose by 30% in individuals that have a single copy of the high-risk allele for the FTO gene, linked with fat mass and obesity, by 67% in those who have two, who averagely gained 3.0 kg (6.6 lb) or more11. With about one sixth of the population of European descent homozygous for this allele, this link between the FTO gene and obesity seems sturdy, but obesity is not all about microbes and genes. A study published in the July 26, 2007 issue of the New England Journal of Medicine, showed that friends play an even greater role in one's risk of obesity more than, for example, do genes12. The researchers refashioned a social network among participants of the Framingham Heart Study that showed the ties between friends, neighbours, spouses, and family members and observed that the risk of someone being obese increased by 171%, if another, a friend, became obese in a given time period. The researchers also noted that the risk of one sibling in a pair of adult siblings being obese rose by 40%, the other sibling obese, and the clustering of obesity in communities, the risk of an obese person's friend's friend being obese, roughly 20%. This was higher in the observed than in a random network, the effect eliminated only by the 4th degree of separation. This study not only has major health policy and public health implications, and would likely interest firms but also highlights the increasing interest in medical circles, and which should be so, in business, in interconnectedness, and the role of networks in health and disease. Indeed, networks, including social networks would become increasingly prominent in health issues, for example, social networks and their effect on the spread of obesity or pathogens, including influenza, severe acute respiratory syndrome (SARS) or the human immunodeficiency virus (HIV) 13. It would also likely interest firms that neural networks also play a major role in various psychiatric and neurodegenerative diseases and that, cellular networks are possible conduits for the propagation of genetic defects to other non-defective genes14. In fact, network medicine research focuses on understanding the links between the cellular, disease, and social networks in the mechanisms of disease causation, among others, including mechanism of drug actions and their side effects, the potential of an appreciation of these processes for firms in achieving the dual healthcare delivery objectives (DHD), self-evident. Indeed, obesity, for example, has associations with seven diseases, including asthma, lipodystrophy, and glioblastoma, and genetic probably explains obesity for firms, in particular depending on whether they have the resources so to do, to employ the services of professionals, for example, syndicated researchers, who would help in presenting to them, the relevant information crucial to factor into the firms' healthcare strategies. As firms, increasingly embrace the need for elucidating their peculiar circumstances, and incorporating novel knowledge and information into their initiatives in health services provision, the benefits accruable from such an orientation would increase even more, including positioning the firms for competitive advantage, not to mention increased profitability. Thus, healthcare would become a strategic asset, its qualitative and cost-effective delivery, potentially, core competence. The efficiency of service provision by firms would not occur by accident, at least not in the main. Given the probability of serendipity, it might, but a direct focus on healthcare issues and the applications of knowledge gained thereof in the design of initiatives that would improve the nature and quality of health services provision would be likelier differentiating among firms in future and more possibly a success driver.

As earlier noted, the acquisition of knowledge could either herald opportunities or portend problems. It would be necessary for firms to tell the difference, an attribute upon which the success of their initiatives would precariously hinge. In fact, the hallmark of a firm that would be able to convert its expenditures on health services provision into competitive advantage would be to do the same whenever possible for what might at first seem to be insurmountable challenges. Thus, it would be one thing to realize that a third of its workforce is obese for example, and in some misguided cases, the firm wanting to impose some regulation that would limit the weight of its workers, for example, prohibiting the sale of pop on its premises. The question is that these workers might drink even more pop at home than they would have at work. A different firm, more attuned to the futility of coercion in changing human behaviour would adopt a different approach, for example, emphasizing the benefits of a cocoa drink, and the need to be aware of the adverse health effects of carbonated drinks, which might actually make its cafeteria sell more drinks, only this time, not pop. Encouraging their workers to exercise, for example, subsidizing their treadmills might also produce the desired results as opposed to issues prohibitions, ultimatums, and threats of job loss for examples. Firms might also buttress the claims that they make in for example memos regarding certain health issues with current research evidence, well-put together by their staff, or contracted out as noted earlier. Such firms would discover that the benefits derivable from such efforts would far outweigh in human and material terms, the costs involved. The idea then is that in weighing the input from developments in the determination of relevant healthcare programs, firms would need to make some amount of financial investments that might seem, on the surface, difficult to rationalize, but which on scrutiny would reveal astuteness in planning and vision for which it would be convinced the initial financial was well worth. In other words, decisions on such investments would constitute a major challenge to some firms, but perhaps in doing so, such firms would learn, not only to appreciate that part of the ingredients of success is the ability to make tough decisions. Furthermore, they would also learn that at the end of the day success means in part having something to show for the decisions, but that decisions regarding health services, a complexity of innumerable hybrid transactions, could not ever be mincemeat. Thus, we see again, how firms' involvement in health services provision could pose a major challenge, but which smart firms could turn into prospects, given the benefits, even albeit in the long term that the decisions taken could confer in improved management terms, including in financial management, on the firms. These are besides those regarding the provision of qualitative and efficient health services for their workers. Our interests here therefore, revolve not around chronicling specific prospects and challenges, but in a somewhat generic sense emphasizing the role that firms' focus on health services could play in generating either, and in addressing both successfully, their origins regardless. We also anticipate that firms would show more interests in these issues, realizing as we attempt to show that it is in their best interests so to do. In countries such as the U.S., current figures do not show that firms are in a sense and in the main, adopting this perspective, many still not involved in health services provision for their workers, particularly the small firms. As figure 1 below sourced from a chart released on September 14, 2007, by The Commonwealth Fund, shows, employers provided health benefits to over 160 million working Americans and their families in 2006, hence a major source of healthcare coverage in the country.

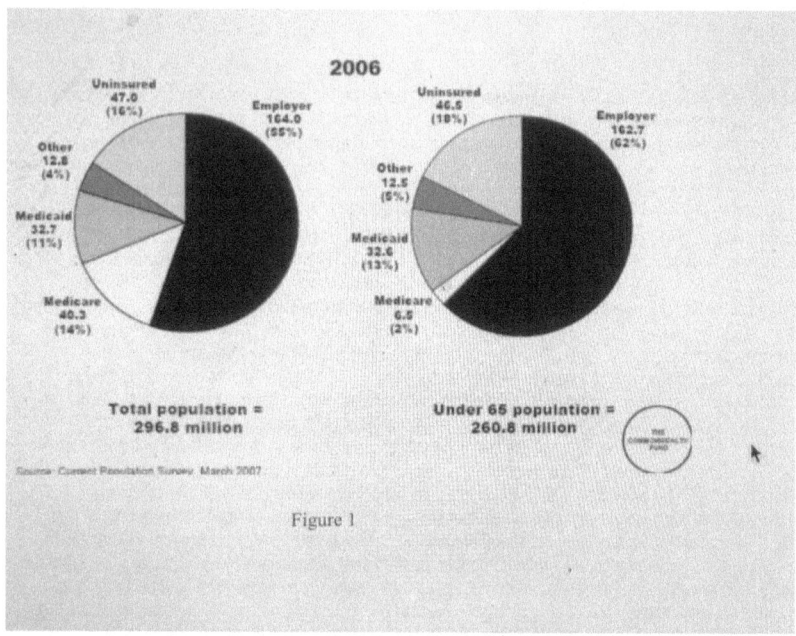

Figure 1

There is also no doubt that the sustained growth in healthcare costs in putting financial pressure of employers and compromising their ability to provide their workers with comprehensive healthcare benefits, despite the substantial health spending by government, which in relation to other countries Figure 2, clearly demonstrates. This figure shows the percentage of National Health Expenditures spent on Insurance Administration and Overhead, in 2003, in several developed countries, the U.S., evidently outspending them all even this restricted domain, but which nonetheless is instructive. It is because it only underscores the point regarding the likely increased participation of employers in health services provision rather than the other way round given the un-sustainability of such massive spending by government on just administration, but also despite the apparent current disinterest among some firms in health services provision.

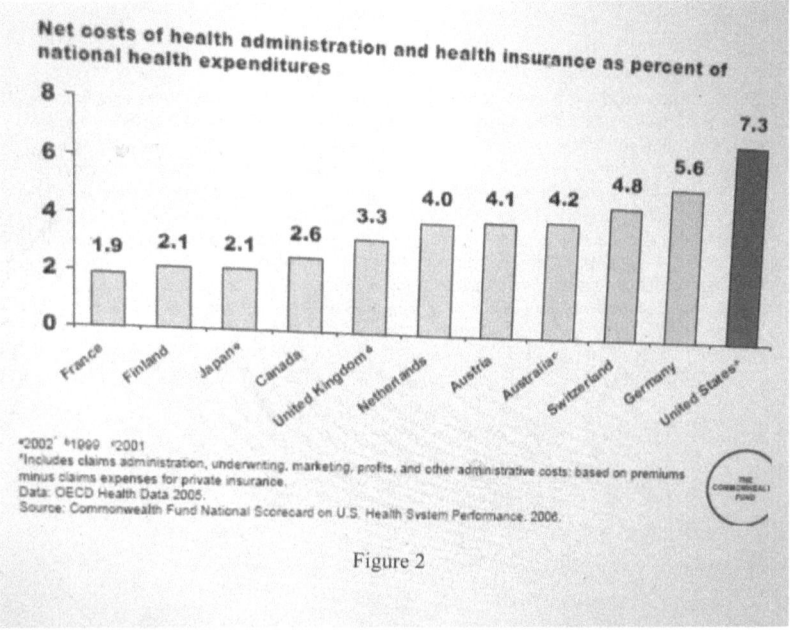

Figure 2

Indeed, despite that, the Commonwealth Fund study charts highlight the fact many Americans are not currently in the employer-sponsored health system, that many deductibles particularly for small firms are increasing as Figure 3 shows, and that most of uninsured adults are in working families, among others, it also noted the importance of employer-sponsored health insurance, which employers are increasingly acknowledging. More employers, even small firms, for example, admit that health benefits are important to staff recruitment and retention for example, as they are to improving workers' health, morale, and satisfaction, and indeed, their performance and productivity. Clearly, the acknowledgement by even small firms of these benefits of health services provision to their workers points to the direction employer-sponsored health insurance heads, even despite its current overall relatively poor showing, in the country. In fact, where hold that this pattern is not likely to occur only in the U.S., but rather worldwide regardless of a country's health financing model. Indeed, one would be hard-pressed to find any country even now that solely finances its health service with public funds, or with private funds. As we saw earlier, the U.S., for example, despite the prominence of employer-sponsored health and private insurance in its health system, depends substantially on the public for some of its healthcare programs such as Medicare and Medicaid.

The likelihood in fact is that employer-sponsored health insurance would increasingly become the prevalent model of health services provision as governments worldwide increasingly realize the futility in becoming involved in health services provision, in the face of ever-increasing healthcare spending despite not so impressive services provision. The reasons for the dearth of commensurate service quality in many health systems are legion, some generic, others specific to the particular health jurisdiction, but the outcome is typically similar: soaring healthcare costs. Among the key challenges that firms would face as they become more engrossed in health services provision therefore would be to ensure that they do not become victims of the very problems, inefficiencies that compromise cost-effectiveness, driving health services provision away from government hands. Indeed, short of asserting that government operations would become more efficient and not bogged down in political expediencies, for instance, firms would have little if any choice but to avoid being victims of these problems. In other words, as firms attune to the issues involved, that for example, it is in their best interests to take the issue of healthcare seriously, so would they, those pertaining to doing so efficiently and cost-effectively. Why would small firms for example not examine Figure 3 and

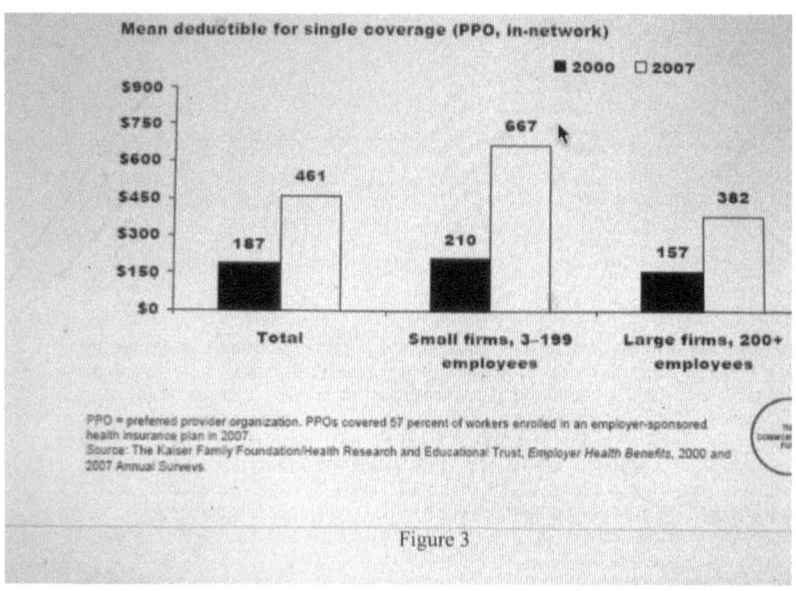

Figure 3

wonder why deductibles are not as high among larger firms and are even falling relatively whereas the reverse is the case with the smaller firms? Could large firms for example be exploiting scale economies, and why could small firms, in alliance with one another not do the same? Here is where the issues we have raised in our discussion such as the freedom of choice and that of the operations of the market come in, regardless of the displeasure of the major health plans, as some would contend, which might drive up the costs of premiums. The point in fact is that the feared essentially shoving-out of the market of smaller health insurers that their won scale economies might cause would be redundant were there in reality such freedom. Given the interests of firms in health services provision that we have here argued would increase in the years ahead, and the likely initiatives that would thereof emanate, predicated on acquiescence to the emerging knowledge that medical and technological progress among others would engender, that freedom would no doubt eventually materialize. The challenge for these firms is in ensuring that it does, which is unlikely going to be much of a challenge given that their interests are at stake. The point is not about firms and their employees driving health plans and insurers or any other player in the healthcare delivery enterprise out of business, but rather the need for and the imperative of improving the efficiency of healthcare transactions, to improve the quality of healthcare delivery. Indeed, it would be in the interest of all players that this happens, none, as in keeping with the underlying principles of free trade, would lose out in the end, in particular within the context of their place not just in the local and national economies but also in the increasingly hyper-competitive global economy. Here again, firms that appreciate in full the interplay of these issues, would recognize the potential of converting the challenge of assuring the autonomy of its workers in decision making regarding their health, rather than coercing them, into immense prospects. Such prospects would likely include those delivered by their workers in terms of commitment to well thought-out healthcare initiatives, and in relation to which, major cost containment for example, and the ability of the firms to achieve the dual healthcare delivery objectives, among others, set out in their healthcare strategies. Our emphasis on the prospects/challenges dyad being in a sense symbiotic highlights an approach to a framework on health services provision by firms that we would likely see increasingly embraced. This is more so as the responsibility for these services, directly or indirectly, as the case may be, broadens the scope of firms in management and operational terms, among others, creating the need for innovation to address elements of the dyad, the learning curve increasingly shorter, meanwhile harnessed in core competencies that confer competitive edge. Yet, it is important that firms achieve a mindset that confers the ability to conceptualize healthcare issues appropriately lest let the opportunity slip by literally to ensure the effective conversion of the issues and experiences accumulating in addressing which for the betterment of the firm. This perhaps would be for many firms, the first challenge, and a key one at that.

References

1. DeNavas-Walt, C.B. Proctor, and C.H. Lee. Income, Poverty, and Health Insurance Coverage in the United States: 2005. U.S. Census Bureau., August 2006.

2. Available at

http://www.cms.hhs.gov/apps/media/press/testimony.asp?Counter=806&int

NumPerPage=10&checkDate=&checkKey=&srchType=1&numDays=3500&srch

Opt=0&srchData=&keywordType=All&chkNewsType=7&intPage=&showAll=

&pYear=&year=&desc=false&cboOrder=date Accessed on July 15, 2007

3. Strunk, Bradley C., and Paul B. Ginsburg. 2003. "Tracking Health Care Costs: Trends Stabilize but Remain High in 2002." Health Affairs web exclusive. http://www.healthaffairs.org, accessed June 11.

4. Haber, SG; Khatutsky, G; Mitchell, JB. 2001. Covering the uninsured through Medicaid: Lessons from Oregon Health Plan. Available at: http://www.cms.hhs.gov/Reports/downloads/haber2_2001_1.pdf Accessed on July 15, 2007

5. Lipson, D.J., and Schrodel, S.P., State-Subsidized Insurance Programs for Low- Income People. Alpha Center. Washington, D.C. November 1996.

6. Office for Oregon Health Plan Policy and Research (OHPPR), The Uninsured in Oregon. Salem, OR. 1999.

7. Zuckerman, Stephen. 2003. "Gains in Public Health Insurance Offset Reductions in Employer Coverage among Adults." Snapshots of America's Families III, No. 8. Washington, D.C.: The Urban Institute.

8. Clemens-Cope, Lisa, et al, Changes in Employees' Health Insurance Coverage, 2001-2005, Kaiser Commission on Medicaid and the Uninsured, October 2006.

9. The Henry J. Kaiser Family Foundation. Employee Health Benefits: 2006 Annual Survey. 26 September 2006.

10. Available at:

http://www.nytimes.com/2006/08/13/magazine/13obesity.html?_r=2&oref=sl

ogin&oref=slogin Accessed on October 8, 2007

11. Frayling TM, Timpson NJ, Weedon MN, et al. A common variant in the FTO gene is associated with body mass index and predisposes to childhood and adult obesity. Science 2007; 316:889-94.

12. Christakis NA, Fowler JH. The spread of obesity in a large social network over 32 years. N Engl J Med 2007; 357:370-9.

13. Barabasi A. Network Medicine-From Obesity to the "Diseaseome". N Engl J Med 2007; 357:404

14. Barabási A-L, Oltvai ZN. Network biology: understanding the cell's functional organization. Nat Rev Genet 2004; 5:101-15

Healthcare Costs Kaleidoscope

Cost sharing in healthcare delivery evokes different reactions in different people. The idea of shifting health care costs is vile to some, a delight to others. In many countries such as the U.S., businesses are reeling under the yoke of soaring healthcare costs and many are desperately seeking ways out. Many in fact, no longer offer healthcare coverage, and those that still do are increasing employee deductibles, co-pays, and premium quotas, for examples. These measures are escalating out-of-pocket healthcare costs to employees understandably to the chagrin of many. Indeed, many would argue that cost-shifting strategies are stopgap solutions to a pervasive problem whose underlying causes are legion, not to mention its solutions, addressing both of which raises questions regarding the nature and extent of government or private sector involvement in so doing. In the U.S for example, a study published in the June 7, 2005 issue of the journal, Health Affairs showed that homogeneous national strategies focused on the uninsured do not generate homogeneous national outcomes[1], with the degree of cross-state variations in uninsurance rates, economic and labor-market indices, and healthcare markets remarkable. The researchers examined this variation by comparing the effects of standard tax credit and Medicaid expansion proposals in different states, and found that some states did well, others not so well under all policies, state effects on uninsurance rates across policies varying by at least a factor of 2.5. Thus, analyses of different health insurance proposals and indeed, other health reform initiatives, in either the public or private sector, need to focus on both their national and states impact, on both of which levels, their short-and long-term ramifications for businesses and for the overall economy could be quite profound. This implies that strategic considerations by firms on healthcare provision need to be generic and specific, as opposed to intrinsically simplistic annual wholesale costs shifting exercises that make little if any dent on curtailing their soaring healthcare budgets. Even if its face validity seemed obtuse, on scrutiny, it belies the crucial need for businesses to examine comprehensively, the interplay of reasons for the escalating healthcare costs in their respective jurisdictions. In developed countries such as the U.S, Canada, and the U.K, for examples, firms need to be cognizant of the impact of aging population on health and economic variables, among others, and to determine the measures actionable. What could a firm do for example, to encourage healthy lifestyles among its employees, which might not only enhance their well being, but also help prevent chronic diseases, in effect, ensuring that it has a healthy and productive workforce, besides reducing health spending? How could the firm contribute to improving the efficiency and quality of health services provision in the country, promote widespread healthcare information and communication technologies (healthcare ICT), reduce the costs associated with expensive, high-tech procedures, and lower health insurance premiums? How could it help reduce service over-utilization and wastage the 'all or none' attitude to service usage that indiscriminate healthcare cost shifting for example, could occasion? Is it in companies' strategic interests that costs sharing discourage, as it does in some instances, the demand for required services? Should firms not be keen to prevent not just absenteeism, but also presenteeism, the latter wherein employees, even those with great job attendance records, work with impairments and disabilities that compromise efficiency? Should this not be more so given that in a 2001 report, "Presenteeism: A Clear View of a Growing Problem," Clark Marcus, of Amacore Group, Inc.,noted presenteeism results in employers losing over 30 times in productivity as from absenteeism, a recent Canadian survey showing that nearly two-thirds of Canadian workers (62%) go to work when mentally and physically ill2? These questions no doubt exemplify the scope of the relevant issues firms need to consider in tackling the perennial healthcare costs increases that they need to contain, simultaneous providing their employees qualitative, accessible, and affordable health services. No doubt, firms would be able to address some of these issues better than they would others, the potential to do so effectively reciprocal to the extent of the problem's specificity or otherwise. Regardless of how much specific or generic the problem is, however, that the firm would need not just to appreciate its nature and ramifications in full, but that of the need to collaborate to a more or less extent with other healthcare stakeholders, for an effective solution to the problem. Thus, a firm would need to appreciate the need for an all-inclusive decomposition/exposition of the issues it has identified as crucial to reducing its healthcare spending while not compromising the quality of care that its employees receive, in embracing, for example, consumer-driven health care (CDHC), versus deductibles and cost-shifting, with their inherent financial obstacles to care. In other words, the firm would not just assume that CDHC would help it reduce health-spending, understanding that it would on the other hand foster rational decision-making on health matters, promoting rather than hindering care receipt, but doing the reverse for service over-utilization and wastage, characteristics with significant cost-containment potential. Even as this approach to healthcare strategy becomes increasingly popular among firms, in the U.S., for example, that they would achieve the desired results hinges on fully appreciating the relevant issues and taking the required measures to ensure its success. Here again, the emphasis is on the eclectic nature of the transactions that constitute healthcare delivery, and the difficulty in their objective measurement, which is crucial, as in performance-based reimbursement of healthcare providers, or indeed, in consensus on service/product pricing, both of which examples could hike or lower costs substantially. That every consumer under CDHC has first-dollar coverage hence obviates concerns about cost barriers could signal the potential for services not optimized, driving up costs, if firms did not take the required measures to address the relevant issues. For example, they need to promote initiatives to reduce, if not eliminate, the seeming information glut that nonetheless is an information chasm or dearth, considering that the healthcare consumer either overwhelmed or lacks the understanding for such information to be valuable in decision making, if it was not entirely nonexistent, essentially lacks it. How would such a healthcare consumer even with CDHC make the right choices regarding service utilization in what for example, some would term a healthcare chimera that pervasive direct-to-consumer media melees ballyhoo? It behooves the firm therefore, to say the least, to factor the efficient and cost-effective provision of the required information to make rational healthcare delivery choices into its healthcare strategy to set the stage, literally for success, to being with, not mention its obligations to its shareholders to remain viable, let alone thrive. It is indeed, the case, that not just employers, but insurers, increasingly recognize the need for such information provision, many deploying extensively, healthcare information and communication technologies (healthcare ICT) to facilitate information dissemination and sharing among healthcare stakeholders. In others words, businesses need also to acknowledge the importance of the cost-effective and efficient transactions involved in healthcare delivery being a key aspect of reducing their healthcare spending, hence the need for choices among healthcare providers for example, with value propositions that create the enabling milieu for this to happen. With regard these technologies for example, maximizing the potential benefits in care delivery and pecuniary terms requires their ubiquity in services domains and among healthcare stakeholders, including the healthcare consumer. Thus, to realize their benefits in full would require closing the information loop, so to say, as any gaps in information transfer between these stakeholders would compromise the effectiveness of the technologies, in improving the quality of care delivered, hence in reducing healthcare costs, hence spending. In making choices regarding plans and providers therefore, firms, would also need to encourage the use of relevant technologies, for example to access health information, and services/products prices, by their employees, and indeed, to be able to play their part, in closing the information transfer loop to which other key healthcare stakeholders contribute appropriate information. Clearly, still on this example, firms, except those directly involved in technology development and provision, and in technology policy-related issues, would have little if anything to do with certain aspects of the diffusion of these technologies, among healthcare stakeholders, for examples standards issues, or privacy and confidentiality legislation. This underscores the need for collaboration between agencies and organizations in the public and private sectors, on these issues. In other words, the need to shelve the 'silo mentality' in approaching healthcare costs and other issues holding back progress in healthcare delivery in many countries is ripe. In particular, businesses cannot afford to be stuck in this mindset as the example of managed care in the U.S failing to reduce their healthcare costs woes, but in fact escalating them, shows. Similarly, embracing CDHC as a fad rather than endeavouring to appreciate its core issues in full and applying the insights gained to addressing identified healthcare costs issues peculiar to the firms is likely a recipe for failure too. Meanwhile, the question of the extent of the elasticity of firms' tolerance for such a state of affairs highlights the urgency of actionable initiatives to avert it, which underscores the nature and extent of employers' involvement in their employees' personal health issues, hitherto essentially shunned to avoid infringing on workers' privacy or accusations of discriminations based on ill-health, among others. Yet, we would likely increasingly see more firms showing more interest in what employees are doing or not doing regarding their health that increase healthcare costs as more employers would devise incentives and penalties as appropriate to keep soaring healthcare costs in check. In short, we would increasingly see employer-sponsored health benefits focused on strategic initiatives aimed specifically at supporting employees to adopt healthy lifestyles and improve their well being, in order to achieve the DHDO and enhance productivity, hence bottom line, rather than simply sharing healthcare costs.

The findings of a recent PricewaterhouseCooper 2007 employer survey3 of over 100 top executives, those that took part in the 2007 and 2005 employer panels with an average of 9,350 employees and $2.13 billion in revenue, overall the firms representing 1.4 million employees across business sectors are instructive. The survey of employer attitudes and healthcare strategies in the U.S, showed that employers, particularly large multinational firms, strongly support employer-sponsored healthcare coverage, 87% of surveyed employers opposed to not doing so altogether. Ninety-four percent of employers considered that there is room for improving current practices regarding supporting their employees in managing their own health to help reduce costs and enhance productivity. The survey also showed that 73 percent of employers believed that retiree health coverage creates financial pressure on firms and needs changing via reducing employer quotas. Sixty-two percent wanted employees with unhealthy lifestyle behaviours to pay a larger share of their health benefits costs, and employers consider offering financial incentives to employees for examples cash for completing health risk appraisals, or agreed-upon goals such as quitting cigarette smoking or losing a given amount of weight. Eighty percent of surveyed employers in 2007, versus 84% in 2006, were convinced that offering financial incentives for employees taking part in healthy lifestyle programs would cut their firm's healthcare costs. Nonetheless, employers would need to be careful not to infringe state and federal laws, or compromise privacy, or discriminate against employees, among others, in implementing these incentives/penalties initiatives, and better still, actually aim to achieve the same goals without coercion. Indeed, regarding the provision of information on quality slashing the company's health care costs, just 62% concurred, which suggests that motivating employees to act on information to change behaviour is going to be just as important as providing health information to begin with in the days ahead. The survey also showed that employers are starting to help employees in managing their own retiree health and related costs. Almost 80% of surveyed employers were in favour of providing savings account mechanisms, tax inducements, and coverage access even if not funded by the employers. The variety of measures that employers would increasingly employ would also predicate more on objective evidence of their benefits in achieving the DHDO. The results of investigations such as a recent study aimed at determining the relationship between body mass index (BMI) (calculated as weight in kilograms divided by height in meters squared) and number and types of workers' compensation claims, associated costs, and lost workdays, are thus likely to be of keen interest to employers4. Among the participants were 11,728 healthcare and university employees (34,858 full-time equivalents [FTEs]) with at least one health risk appraisal. The results showed an obvious direct relationship between BMI and rate of claims, the BMI effect patent in work injury, or illness that pertained to most parts of the body, sprain or strain, contusion or bruise, and pain and inflammation, the key BMI effects drivers. Claims regarding the back; wrist, or arm; neck or shoulder; and lower extremity (knee, foot, and hip) were also common and significantly linked to BMI category. However, BMI most significantly affected claims resulting from lifting, falls or slips, and exertion. The study also showed that employees in obesity class III (BMI =40) had 11.65 claims per 100 FTEs, recommended-weight employees, 5.80. The researchers also noted an even stronger effect on lost workdays (183.63 compared to 14.18 lost workdays per 100 FTEs), medical claims costs ($51,091compared to $7,503 per 100 FTEs), and indemnity claims costs ($59,178 compared to $5,396 per 100 FTEs). It is clear from the previously mentioned examples that companies would be examining the diverse causes of healthcare costs, and taking more objective cost-containment measures, and emphasis would be on the increasing role of the employee in achieving this goal. However, this focus would be likelier all-inclusive, the interplay of the various factors that impinge on not just the employee, but also the firms, healthcare providers, suppliers, and insurers, among other healthcare stakeholders, going to be of legitimate and likely increasing interests in any effort to contain healthcare costs. A recent Commonwealth Fund scorecard, released on June 13, 2007, on the performance indicators measures in the U.S.attests to the need for such comprehensive understanding of the issues involved in potential variations in healthcare costs among states, for example, for companies to be able to achieve their costs-cutting goals, among others5. Aimed at following the National Scorecard on U.S. Health System Performance, published in 2006, the State Scorecard evaluated state variation across key dimensions of health system performance, namely, access, quality, avoidable hospital use and costs, equity, and healthy lives, wide variation among states noted. The report also noted the potential for substantial improvement in terms of access, quality, costs, and lives, for examples highlighted were all states to approach levels achieved by the leading states namely Hawaii, Iowa, New Hampshire, and Vermont. The leading states consistently outperformed lagging states such as Oklahoma, Mississippi, Texas, and Arkansas, which finished at the bottom, on multiple indicators and dimensions. The report noted that if all states did as well as the top performers, the country would have 90 000 fewer deaths before age 75 years yearly, 22 million adults and children now lacking health insurance coverage would have coverage, and Medicare could save up to $22 billion per year. Firms contemplating healthcare strategies would be keen to know that states with the lowest rates of uninsured residents scored highest on preventive and chronic disease care measures, and other quality indicators, and that the study showed no systematic link between care cost and care quality. The report, Aiming Higher, also indicates that states with higher medical costs seemed to have higher rates of potentially preventable hospital use, for examples, high admission rates for complications from chronic conditions such as diabetes, and asthma. It also notes there is room for improvement in standards even in the best-performing states. Thus, only 65% of adults with diabetes received recommended preventive care services in Hawaii, the state that scored the highest score for this indicator, only 50% of individuals aged 50 years or older, receiving all recommended screening and preventive care in highest ranked state, Minnesota. There is no doubt that firms would benefit from understanding the complex interplay of variables that determine health and disease, to enable them formulate objective healthcare strategies that would result in the achievement of the twin objectives mentioned earlier of qualitative healthcare provision for their workers simultaneously reducing costs. Indeed, for them to have such understand would require familiarity with developments in particular in medicine, and allied fields from which clear strategic objectives could emanate consistent with the sometimes-paradigmatic shifts in these fields that nonetheless have profound impact on medical practice, and indeed, on health practices by individuals that would improve their health and well being. An example of such developments is the emergence from research recently that obesity is socially contagious[6]. To appreciate fully the ramifications of this finding, consider an earlier US study that showed compared the effects of obesity, overweight, smoking, and problem drinking on healthcare use and health status based on national survey data, and showed that obesity outranks both drinking and smoking in its adverse effects on health and healthcare costs[7]. The study showed that obesity has about the same link with chronic health conditions, as does twenty years' aging, which far exceeds the links of smoking or problem drinking. The study also showed that utilization and health effects correspond, obesity linked with a 36 percent increase in inpatient and outpatient spending and a 77 percent increase in medications, versus a 21 percent increase in inpatient and outpatient spending and a 28 percent increase in medications for current smokers and smaller effects for problem drinkers. These findings are at odds with the more consistent focus in recent decades on drinking and smoking in not just clinical practice, but also in public health policy, and suggest a redirection in focus, in these areas from which firms could take a cue in formulating appropriate healthcare strategies. This is more so considering that the three conditions are known risk factors for chronic health conditions, such as cancer, diabetes, or heart disease, themselves primary drivers of health care spending, disability, and death, and in particular as although they are all still relatively prevalent, obesity is even more so in recent times.

Overweight and obesity, increased amounts of body fat, commonly evaluated by the body-mass index (BMI, being weight in kilograms divided by height in meters squared) are increasingly global problems. According to the standard criteria of having a BMI of less than 18.5 being underweight, of 18.5–24.9, normal, of 25–29.9, overweight, and of 30 or more obese, about one in three Americans are overweight, although not obese, and a further one in five, obese[8,9,10]. Despite that BMI does not accurate differentiate fat mass from lean mass, hence misclassifies some individuals, and that researchers employ other measures such as waist circumference, waist-to-hip ratio, and skin-fold thickness, especially in epidemiological studies, BMI is still a valuable index of overweight/obesity and the health problems associated with them. Thus, there is an association between a higher BMI, starting in the upper end of the normal weight category, with increased mortality and higher risk for coronary heart disease (CHD), high blood pressure, osteoarthritis, diabetes mellitus, and some forms of cancer[11, 12,

13, 14. The point is that even modest weight reductions could substantially increase one's lifespan, something that many firms would deem serious enough to warrant being of significance for their healthcare strategies, and initiatives arising thereof, and justifiably so. Given the potential to achieve weight reduction inexpensively, relative to the enormous health benefits this would in turn yield, we would likely see firms exploring the variety of options to promote weight loss among their workers voluntarily. This they would in fact also regarding other preventable risk factors for many of the chronic diseases common in particular among individuals as they become older. Would firms also not be keen for example to know why in the U.S. for example, the increase in overweight, and including obesity between 1960 and 1980 was just minimal, as opposed to the dramatic increases recent times, increases mostly in the obese category, which recorded a growth of 60% just between 1991 and 200010? Is a change in diet responsible, or it that more food is available or that certain types of food, specifically 'junk food', is more available, or is its marketing that is more aggressive? Are people spending more time indoors, watching TV, and not exercising enough, or are there emotional factors involved driving gluttony? The answers to such questions would in future constitute legitimate quests by firms seeking to develop the appropriate healthcare strategies for their workers, as these answers could be invaluable in the constituents of the strategies and the initiatives emanating thereof. The future of firms would be tied to that of the health of their workers more than ever before as employer-sponsored health insurance becomes more pervasive, and it becomes clear that its role in the health system of any country, its health financing system regardless, would be indeed, pivotal. Firms would also be more interested to know about developments in the medical field in many different respects, for example, clinical, legal, and regulatory, among others, as these could be far-reaching not just for the success of their healthcare strategies but their implementation to start with. Thus, they would be keen to know the outcome of the debate on whether obesity is a disease or disability, recognition of which disease paradigm with potent ramifications for health insurance coverage, parity legislation, taxation of weight loss programs, and healthcare costs, among others, a move that the American Obesity Association and other advocacy groups, endorse. Indeed, there have been many instances in which groups of individuals advocate for considerations of other conditions as diseases, which if successful would expand the list that firms would need to be watchful of the resulting changes as they could have significant effects on their healthcare strategies. It is thus clear, that firms would need to have a broad-based approach to conceptualizing healthcare costs, as the dimensions of the healthcare delivery enterprise whose inefficient operations, if it needed exist at all, could have significant cost implications would become ever more, legitimate matters for attention. In other words, cost drivers would not necessarily imply the use, some would contend, wasteful use, of expensive technologies, or of poly-pharmacy, when not treating different conditions, and in fact using, sometimes medications in the same pharmacological category to treat the same condition or symptoms. Rather, firms would be keen on details on the transactions involved in disease management, and in improving its efficiency and cost effectiveness, in other words, not only in outcomes, but in the processes resulting in these outcomes too. This would require embarking on analyzing issues, and processes, for example via process cycle analysis, the resulting decomposition/exposition, the starting point for the objective understanding of the pertinent issues that are hiking transactions costs. Thus, in conducting such analyses, firms, determining the role that a lack of commitment to the value propositions of a healthcare provider, health plans, or others in the healthcare delivery chain, would not end there, but followed up with the require actions. Thus, it might mean that the healthcare provider needs to implement a certain healthcare information and communication technology (healthcare ICT), to improve certain processes to bring transaction costs down, something, which the firm would be, prepared to point out, and upon which, if the reaction of the provider were inadequate, the firm might need to take additional measures. Firms would have to be proactive in addressing the many issues it could and should follow through with the answers to its questions that its various analyses reveal. The reasons for firms taking such measures would be clear as they accept the facts of the imperative of employer-sponsored health insurance in the overall health insurance scheme of things, literally. Because their workers are at the core of this imperative, which essentially, is the likely increase in the use of this type of insurance firms would in effect ensure that they receive qualitative and cost-effective health services. Yet, and as part of the open-mindedness we mentioned earlier, firms would need to look farther than the immediate to appreciate the obstacles in the ways, some of the issues, seemingly outside their purview that are driving healthcare costs sky-high, but which nonetheless they would have to address. One such issue in the U.S., for example, is that each state disallows its residents buying health insurance coverage across its borders, which gives them a monopoly that they in fact enforce by law, but which drives health insurance premiums up by as much as 15% according the Congressional Budget Office15. Firms might have to lobby Congress to legislating against the ban on out-of-state coverage purchase by workers and their firms, which would slash premiums costs drastically, perhaps, as market forces modulate prices, making health insurance more affordable, and coverage more widespread. There are also dimensions relating to issues with the pharmaceutical industry that firms might need to engage in, to ensure that they achieve the dual healthcare delivery objectives (DHDO), which many firms would see with time, as crucial to their survival, and indeed, progress. In short, and as we have here noted, firms would increasingly appreciate the need to be conversant with these issues, many of which would emerge from the process cycle analyses in which they would engage, and in fact to tackle them appropriately. It might seem superfluous to expect firms to take on these wide-ranging issues just to pay less for healthcare services for their workers. However, the point is that the overriding issue is far deeper in essence than that of money, not to mention the fact that their workers would also save money, and that saving money is only one aspect of the DHDO. The key issue here is that the employer would be playing an increasingly central role in health services provision, and it has to do a great job, literally. That it must is an imperative that is not a whim, but borne out of the reasons it would playing such a pivotal role in the first place, reasons that would drive health services out of government hands and why businesses cannot afford to make the same mistakes to avoid compromising health service provision. Finally, they cannot afford to compromise health services provision because they would jeopardizing their very existence doing so. Thus, the requirements for efficiency would itself be dual, in the main, rooted in responsibility and self-preservation, the former in fact, an enforced element of the first in some instances, even if it need not be. In other words, firms have a duty to their workers to ensure that they receive qualitative and affordable health services, having inherited this responsibility from government essentially bungling their roles, which in fact, should not be their role anyway. They also would benefit in showing that responsibility as their workers become healthier and more productive. It is uncertain though how many firms consider matters this way, but it unlikely that those that would stand any chance to survive would take much longer to begin to appreciate the importance of embracing the achievement of the DHDO as critical goals in, and taking the necessary measures to provide the workers the opportunities for qualitative health services provision. recent study that examines the patterns and prevalence of multiple chronic diseases among Medicaid beneficiaries underscores these points16. The study, published by the Centre for Health Care Strategies, which also examines how better appreciation of such patterns could result in the development of 'more appropriate guidelines, care models, performance measurement systems and reimbursement methodologies for Medicaid' found that beneficiaries with three or more chronic conditions are responsible for a considerable portion of Medicaid spending. That this finding, points to the need for reconsidering care management approaches for high-need, high-cost beneficiaries with many chronic diseases, and that firms could benefit from attention to it, in stemming healthcare costs is not in doubt. Thus, in recognition of the complexity of the management of these chronic conditions, firms, in tackling chronic diseases among their workers, would also have to accept that customary single-disease management programs would likely be inadequate, despite the preliminary appearance of higher costs addressing this complexity. The point in fact is that ultimately, it would likely be more expensive ultimately, ignoring the complex needs of these beneficiaries, and not developing integrated and coordinated healthcare delivery systems that combine clinical care with behavioural and non-medical supportive services for examples10. Firms in many developed countries and not just the U.S., would need to pay attention to this issue over time, given the aging populations of these countries, and the healthcare costs implications of this demographic pattern. Coupled with the fact that many of the countries, lacking manpower, are extending the retirement age, which means that firms would still have on their payrolls perhaps many more individuals with multiple chronic diseases in the years ahead. With over 60 percent of adult Medicaid enrolees having a chronic or disabling condition even now, there could be no gainsaying the matter, in particular as the approach to managing their conditions currently is fragmented, and needlessly expensive, costing as much as 80 percent of state Medicaid budgets17. Thus, firms would increasingly need to devise the means to provide their high-need, high-cost workers with qualitative healthcare without incurring avoidable costs, which highlights the importance of these firms adopting the appropriate healthcare strategies to address issues that are relevant to their peculiar circumstance. These might include, for example, investing in healthcare information and communications technologies (healthcare ICT), and in any other measures that the process cycle analyses they need to conduct would reveal, to ensure that they achieve the stated goals. The point therefore is that firms would be approaching healthcare costs issues differently in the years ahead, in particular in a generic manner, examining the basic elements and issues that drive costs, in a bottom-up fashion, thus ensuring that they did not miss out any pertinent cost driver. In addition to costs, they would also be keen to ensure that the health services that their workers receive are comprehensive, and qualitative, which themselves would reduce morbidities, and ultimately, costs. Healthcare delivery would be different in many respects as employer- sponsored health insurance gains increasing currency, the onus increasingly on firms to take it further along this new path of quality improvement and accountability, one which would focus, in the main, and at all levels, on the realization of the dual healthcare delivery objectives, which in effect would be imperative.

References

1. Glied S, Gould D. Variations In The Impact Of Health Coverage Expansion Proposals Across States Health Affairs Web Exclusive, June 7, 2005

2. Available at: http://www.nupge.ca/news_2006/n06jn06a.htm Accessed on July 22, 2007

3. Tailoring the Approach: Employer Attitudes and Healthcare Strategies Address Distinct Issues. Medical Benefits. 7/15/2007, Vol. 24 Issue 13, p5-8, 3p

4. Truls Ostbye, MD, PhD, et al., Archives of Internal Medicine, April 23, 2007

5. Available at:

http://www.commonwealthfund.org/publications/publications_show.htm?doc _id=494551 Accessed on July 24, 2007

6. Christakis NA, Fowler JH. The spread of obesity in a large social network over 32 years. N Engl J Med 2007; 357:370-9.

7. Sturm R. The Effects Of Obesity, Smoking, And Drinking On Medical Problems And Costs. Health Affairs, March/April 2002; 21(2): 245-253 Available at: http://content.healthaffairs.org/cgi/content/abstract/21/2/245 Accessed on July 21, 2007

8. National Center for Health Statistics, Health, United States, 2000 (Hyattsville,

Md.: NCHS, 2000), Table 69.

9. Flegal KM, et al., "Overweight and Obesity in the United States: Prevalence and Trends, 1960–1994," International Journal of Obesity and Related Metabolic Disorders 22, no. 1 (1998): 39–47.

10. Mokdad AL, et al., "The Spread of the Obesity Epidemic in the United States, 1991–1998", Journal of the American Medical Association 282, no. 16 (1999): 1519– 1522.

11. Field AE, et al., "Impact of Overweight on the Risk of Developing Common Chronic Diseases during a Ten-Year Period," Archives of Internal Medicine 161, no. 13 (2001): 1581–1586

12. National Task Force on the Prevention and Treatment of Obesity, "Overweight, Obesity, and Health Risk," Archives of Internal Medicine 160, no. 7 (2000): 898–904.

13. World Health Organization, Obesity: Preventing and Managing the Global Epidemic, Report of a WHO Consultation, Geneva, 3–5 June 1997 (Geneva: WHO, 1998).

14. Must A et al., "The Disease Burden Associated with Overweight and Obesity", Journal of the American Medical Association 282, no. 16 (1999): 1523–1529;

15. Available at: http://www.cato.org/pub_display.php?pub_id=8715 Accessed on October 8, 2007

16. Kronick et al., "The Faces of Medicaid II: Recognizing the Care Needs of People With Multiple Chronic Conditions," October 2007. Available at: http://www.chcs.org/publications3960/publications_show.htm?doc_id=540806 Accessed on October 8, 2007

17. Available at:

http://www.chcs.org/publications3960/publications_show.htm?doc_id=317310 Accessed on October 8, 2007

The Line-in-Loop Corporate Healthcare Strategy

A recent five-year study of 1,850 companies revealed two key strategies that enable some firms maintain yearly profitability: they expand their core business into an adjacent space, and embark on such expansion in predictable, repeatable ways1, repeatability, in shifting geographic markets, customer segments, product categories, or hybrids of these approaches, among others, doubling success rates among the firms studied. The study also found that firms that succeeded with repeatability showed discipline, screening opportunities robustly before any adjacency move, garnering thereby learning-curve payback, for instance, enhanced strategic clarity, decision-making, simplicity, and speed. The firms also developed their repeatable formulas, keenly interested in and understanding their customers' needs, preferences, and expectations. Yet, corporations cannot ignore the complexity of the interactions of a number of variables including competitive and geopolitical interplays, technical innovation, consumer preferences and capital market swings, and indeed, human capital and labor relations, among others, which affect markets, spewing opportunities and threats, over which management has little if any control. This calls into question the traditional linear, plan then execute, approach to strategy, which no doubt, compromises a firm's ability to incorporate into initiatives the steady flow of information the many variables that impact it generate, a crucial element of the success of its strategies. It thus, underscores the need for firms to be more eclectic in sourcing the ingredients for their strategic orientations. In other words, to ask among others, at what point they should transition from a linear to an iterative mindset, to the loop2, from the line or indeed, to a line-in-loop strategic model, or any other. What is key is that inherent in any model should be the assumption of the imperative of change. In other words, firms need to recognize the potential effects of changes occurring in the many variables that impinge on their businesses on the success or otherwise of their strategies. This means that they should consider every strategy as ongoing work, subject to change, which the interplay of the variables impels. Hence, firms would need to embrace the concept of process cycle analysis, whose rudiments encapsulate that of the strategy loop, and its different iterations. In the equally iterative exposition/decomposition exercises that constitute such analyses would emerge a fuller appreciation of the issue in question, a revelation of the options on the appropriate and non-appropriate measures to take, the approaches to actualizing the measures or otherwise, and the evaluative initiatives required based on novel data and information brought on by further changes. The benefit generically, to a firm of viewing these various aspects of process cycle analysis as process interplays themselves is the elucidating comprehensively, the constituents of success of its strategy, on the one hand, and its construct validity, in the first place, on the other. As a general principle in risk management, firms consider price or market risk, and count on linear risk mitigation in the main, although in practice, besides price uncertainty, many other factors create business risk for example, inputs/outputs-related, demand and supply uncertainty, better addressed via non-linear derivatives, hence again, the wisdom in considering a corporate healthcare strategy formulation does another study mentioned earlier, published in the July 26, 2007 issue of the New England Journal of Medicine, pose that shows that friends play an even more significant role in an individual's risk of becoming obese than do genes3? The researchers, who recreated a social network among participants of the Framingham Heart Study, found the link between friends, neighbours, spouses, and family members and obesity to be remarkable, noting that the risk of someone becoming obese rose by 171%, if another, a friend, became obese in a specified time period. The researchers also found that the risk of one sibling in a pair of adult siblings becoming obese rose by 40%, the other obese, and observed clustering of obesity in communities, the risk of an obese person's friend's friend being obese, roughly 20%, the effect higher in the observed than in a random network. With the FTO gene variant relatively common in human populations, about one in six of white Europeans carrying two copies of the gene variant1, a third of American adults obese, an estimated 2 billion people worldwide, obese or overweight, and about 20 million children under 6, according to the World Health Organization (WHO), the issue indeed, calls for concern. It also exemplifies the fluidity of knowledge of health issues that makes a strictly linear corporate healthcare strategic orientation questionable. Indeed, it stresses the importance of companies, in addressing healthcare issues, to be cognizant of medical progress, which could have profound influence on not just the conceptualization of diseases, but also their management, with potential cost implications likely to interest the healthcare consumer, payers, providers, and indeed, all healthcare stakeholders. The study on the 'spread' of obesity by social networks for example, highlights the growing interest in medicine in the idea of interconnectedness and the role of networks in health and disease. In fact, networks, including social networks would likely gain more prominence in health issues. Social networks and their effect on the spread of obesity or pathogens, including influenza, severe acute respiratory syndrome (SARS) or the human immunodeficiency virus (HIV) would become increasingly, practice, research, and public policy issues5. Other forms of networks, for example, neural networks, also play a major role in diverse psychiatric and neurodegenerative diseases and cellular networks are potential conduits for the transmission of genetic defects to otherwise normal genes6. Indeed, as noted earlier, from network medicine research, with its focus on revealing the associations between the cellular, disease, and social networks in the mechanisms of the origins of disease, and of drug actions and their side effects, among others, could emerge novel paradigms of medical practice. It is thus likely, that firms would show increasing interests in the multilevel-cellular, disease, and social networks that underpin diseases such as obesity, as key elements of their healthcare strategic approaches. This would be even more as research increasingly shows that large number of genes shared by frequently quite unlike disorders not only suggests that they have common genetic origins, but also the need for re-conceptualizing diseases, hence their taxonomy, and management, all of which the corporate world could least afford to ignore. In other words companies intent on achieving the dual healthcare delivery objectives (DHDO), of the provision of accessible and qualitative health services to their workers, health spending not soaring, if actually not falling, would seek the most cost-effective and efficient means of achieving these goals, failure to achieve which, ignoring medical progress, would probably amount. Thus, each firm would need to determine the right mix of linear and loop strategic approaches to employ based on considerations of not just the medical, but also other variables whose interplay could affect its ability to achieve the DHDO directly or otherwise in either a positive or negative way. That such decisions are difficult belies the potential for their lack to create immense financial strain on firms that could result in other measures from which neither the firms nor their workers could benefit even in the short term, hence the critical, and indeed, urgent nature of the decisions.

Firms would also increasingly need to predicate their healthcare strategies on developments in the healthcare and related markets. No doubt, many of these developments follow medical research findings for example, the ever louder clamour by some for the withdrawal of Avandia (Rosiglitazone

Maleate,) the popular anti-diabetic medication from the market due to an increased risk of heart attack. US Food and Drug Administration (FDA) scientist, Dr David Graham, on July 30, 2007, echoed and justified this call to FDA advisors, contending the drug offers no short-term benefits in controlling blood glucose anyway7. Officials of GlaxoSmithKline PLC, which makes Avandia, disputed the studies that showed an increased risk of heart attacks in persons on the drug, insisting that the drug caused few myocardial infarctions. The FDA advisors apparently weighed arguments from both sides and ruled that the medication remains on the market, at least for the time being, although the FDA might eventually reject/accept this advice. Firms would no doubt be increasingly interested in medications and/ or medical procedures, and their potential adverse effects, some of which might be substantial, in pecuniary and disease-burden terms. These issues highlight the fluidity that would characterize strategic approaches in the future considering the pressures from different directions firms would face for instance, to ensure continued profitability of the firms, comply with regulations, and meet the welfare expectations of their employees, including healthcare provision, directly or otherwise, among others. That strategy would be in a perpetual state of flux would be in keeping with the state of affairs in the contemporary zeitgeist. However, so would it be in relation to this state, an increasing appreciation by all concerned of the fundamentals of the interdependencies of a variety of factors in ensuring the survival of the status quo, and in effect, in creating the enabling milieu for it to advance. The persistence to a more or less extent of human capital in the business equation for example would impel the need to eschew any tendency to discountenance it, at least from the perspective of the delivery of labor, be it in a physical or intellectual sense. In other words, even given the technological advances that could threaten in some societies, the tenacity of human capital, human beings would still feature prominently in the scheme of the various systems being operational as required for the perpetuation of life, as we know it. Thus, firms would not yet be giving up on considerations of the strategic approaches to ensuring the efficient and cost-effective operations therein crucial to the firms' very existence, regardless from which of supply or demand perspective, one views the issues involved. It would be the case for example that not just might the chronically ill worker lack the health to take his family on that vacation to the Bahamas they had dreamed of for years, the funds saved up for it might perhaps be those used to settle some unplanned medical bills. The need for an all-inclusive approach to healthcare strategy conceptualization becomes clear, given the stakes of firms in the variety of factors that could impinge on not just their employees' health, but in fact, the 'health' of the firms, as individual firms, and in connection with others, in determining the health or otherwise of the entire economy. To underscore the inadequacy of severing strategy formulation from implementation implicit in the strictly linear approach to strategy with regard healthcare issues, if not any, for that matter, consider the difficulty predicting type 2 diabetes using fasting blood sugar. A research study published in the Oct. 6, 2005 issue of The New England Journal of Medicine 8found that fasting blood sugar levels, now considered normal might in fact be predictive of diabetes someone otherwise healthy. The researchers also found that higher albeit normal blood sugar levels might, in association with body weight, family history of diabetes, or blood triglyceride levels, might point to diabetes. Essentially, therefore, blood sugar levels normal for someone might be abnormal for another, calling the validity of current cut-off points of normal blood sugar into question.This means that firms would need to be cautious in using those values as yardsticks in healthcare strategy, for examples, in recommendations for reward-based preventive health programs, in which many firms increasingly engage, in determining risk for developing diabetes, and in diagnosis of type-2 diabetes. In effect, firms would need to consider the use of fasting blood sugar levels in these and other instances singly, with researches such as this indicating that these levels are inadequate without considerations of family history of diabetes, obesity, cigarette smoking, inactive lifestyle, family history, and other risk factors for diabetes, too, for the individual. The study's findings also have implications for decisions on when to commence treatment for at-risk persons, with potentially significant cost implications. Practice direction is likely going to be more personalized, and given the potential to prevent diseases, some of which, such as diabetes, could become chronic, and result in others such as heart diseases, the increased accuracy in risk determination that this approach engenders would no doubt be attractive to firms in their approach to healthcare strategy. Thus, as opposed to the formulate-and-then-implement approach to strategy, not only would the readiness to incorporate novel information make such distinct stepwise approach to strategy difficult, it would become increasingly clear the prospects derivable in its flexibility, the strategy able to detour in a loop so to speak, to any portion of its prior linear aspects. In other words, even as actions follow formulations, they would need to be maneuverable to ensure that the firm is not overly pursuing strategy, even deemed patently flawed given new information, and change. There is no doubt that firms would be more inclined to pursue the dual healthcare delivery objectives (DHDO) mentioned earlier, but would unlikely achieve these goals stuck with healthcare strategies that are dated, or inapplicable to the health issues, generic and peculiar to the firms, which the strategy should address. This is so even if it were therefore, likely that, firms would increasingly engage the required services to ensure the appropriate strategies are operational. This is an admission of the complexity of the task of applying new information in medicine and indeed, other fields to strategy formulation. Yet, the significance of healthcare strategy for the success of the other strategies of any firm would increasingly justify such moves. In other words, companies need to be able to reasonably project into the long-term, the ramifications of the resource allocations they make now regarding strategic initiatives, including healthcare provision for their workers. It would be near impossible to judge the health status and productivity of their workforce in the future for example, given the context of strategic initiatives, regardless of how crude the estimates are, without considering such information as could help reduce the uncertainty expected with such exercises. In other words, firms can no longer afford to operate ex-post, when in fact the potential for substantial savings while simultaneously ensuring health services provision is real, given attendance to utilizing the necessary tools, for example, process cycle analysis, and the appropriate strategic approaches, for ex-ante determinations. The healthcare field is not the traditional turf of many managers, who would therefore, be taking the best step, intrinsically, to involve an expert in the field in discussions on the potential impact of developments in medicine on a company's healthcare strategy. Thus, contributions to understanding the intricacies of the issues that could constitute elements of the strategy should be eclectic in origin, hence include contributions from representative elements of the company, and possibly an outside expert in medicine. This would ensure that the crucial decomposition exercises that constitute the precedents to exposing other salient issues and the solutions desired, is smooth, and indeed, fruitful. It would become evident for example, why a firm needs to initiate a certain program, for example, chronic disease management. This might involve investments say in the healthcare information and communications technologies (healthcare ICT) that would enable incorporating their workers' personal health records (PHR) systems into the firm's network, to facilitate real-time communications with their doctors, even when mobile, outside the company premises. The firm would be able to estimate ex-ante, the potential benefits of these investments, based among others, on the discussions involving not just management, but healthcare expert, and input, for example from the shop floor, which could also point to the likely acceptance or otherwise of the program by the end-user, the workers. Thus, crucial to every stage of the decomposition of the issues involved is the coalition of sources actively engaged in their determination in the first place, and in breaking them down into further parts in a linear motion, each process, constitutive of elements of the iterative loop emergent with novel data and information that the decomposition/exposition exercises reveal. This is the concept of the line-in-loop strategy approach that firms engaged in formulating a healthcare vision for their workers would increasingly find appropriate in the years ahead, in particular considering what some would deem the feverish pace of medical and technological progress, which promises to be even faster and more complex imminently.

One basis of the line-in-loop approach to healthcare strategy is in the incremental, epiphenomenal nature of scientific, including medical knowledge. It is thus, important not just to examine which of cognitive or drug therapy is preferable for the treatment of depression, and if indeed, treatment should involve both, and to what extent, the differences in treatment outcomes that management is looking at between two providers might have to do with for example medication-dosing practices, with significant cost implications. These costs might not necessarily be those saved because of faster recovery, but might be those that offset such costs due to increased side-effects prevalence rates, which in effect increase morbidity9. In other words, firms would also keenly examine for example a recent UK systematic review of the literature on clinical, utility and cost data, and on relative costs/ benefits decision analysis of antidepressants with cognitive plus medication therapy for moderate, and severe depression in secondary care9. Thus, firms would likely pay attention to the fact that the progression of medical research could be from determining which of cognitive or drug therapy is more effective in the treatment of depression to their adverse effects, and their costs implications, among others, in this instance. Indeed, that this study showed that combination therapy would likely be a cost-effective first-line secondary care treatment for severe but not moderate depression would thus be doubtless instructive, the potential benefits of combination therapy in resource optimization, hence costs containment, yet effective service provision, elements of the DHDO, a strategy firms would increasingly likely pursue. Of significance of this stepwise evolution of scientific knowledge for corporate healthcare strategy is therefore, in anticipating the issues that might feature and to what extent, in future healthcare considerations, their potential cost implications, and impact on the future of the firm. Thus, our understanding of the FTO gene mentioned earlier, currently in relation to obesity might inform considerations of its future role in healthcare initiatives for workers current and future who carry one or both alleles of the gene. This does not necessarily mean that companies would be screening workers for this gene, but might base their initiatives on population prevalence obtained from HapMap, the halotype map of human genome of the International HapMap Project, although avoiding being deemed stereotyping. Yet, firms would also need to be cognizant in their consideration of the incremental nature of the evolution of scientific knowledge concerns regarding it, for example of Thomas Kuhn's queries of the validity of scientific inquiry, in particular the conundrums posed by grounding the normative in the positive10. In highlighting the confounding influence of the 'philosophic value' inherent in the epiphenomena in the so-called 'normal' science, such queries question the validity of the evolution that is a product of the admixture of truth and value as the example of the opposition by the zeitgeist of the requests of certain British scientists recently to breed a human/cow hybrid. This was despite that these scientists affirmed that the studies would help in elucidating the pathophysiology of some diseases, and facilitate novel drug-therapy developments. Such opposition no doubt raises questions about its disruption to the incremental knowledge acquisition in this knowledge domain, hence of whether the redirection of incremental knowledge thereof, still makes the domain 'normal science.' Thus, does the opposition not essentially constitute the grounding of value in truth, the redirection in knowledge acquisition resulting not in incremental 'truth' knowledge but say, 'value-on-truth'? Thus, even science inquiry is fundamentally flawed, and indeed, in The Structure of Scientific Revolutions (SSR) (1962) Kuhn argued that science does not progress via a linear new knowledge accretion, but rather features periodic revolutions he termed 'paradigm shifts.' Indeed, events in the real world do not always proceed linearly, but rather characterized also by convolutions, and as what Japanese strategists term the strategic triangle, that is the interplay of the business corporation, the customer, and the competition essentially slug it out, with often uncertain outcomes, strategic thinking should not also expect to be linear. Rather, it should be flexible, line-in-loop, agile enough to steer along the appropriate path as events unfold. There is no doubt that the mass flight cancellations by the NW Airlines in the US in late July 2007 would have had damaging effects on the carrier's purse and patronage. Yet, the explanation, at least one of them, that shortage of pilots, many calling in sick, would require not just attention to the healthcare needs of the pilots, but also to their conditions of service, including the pecuniary aspects. These issues, whose appropriate solutions would unlikely be, the result of a linear strategy would on the other hand, be line intermingled with loop approaches in a veritable mix of creativity, intuition, and rationality, amicable to management and the pilots' union, for example. Thus, an enterprising strategist might examine the ramifications of the increasingly customer-centric business milieu, for example, for healthcare strategy formulation/implementation. This might be not just in relation to the company's workers being customers themselves, of health plans and providers, and what the workers could expect to receive in terms of health services, but also the workers as the effective links between the business corporation and its customers and what value propositions it could offer the latter. Thus, such might inform strategic considerations, for example, for retailer that might consider incorporating on its premises, a health and fitness gym, where both its workers and customers could work-out, even if it were just tapping the floor to play computer games for a few minutes, mentally and physically, or a snoozing room, for periodic power naps. Such initiatives might enhance total customer value for the company, simultaneously keeping its workers healthier, thus enhancing their productivity, and thereby further increasing the firm's prospects of achieving its value propositions to its customers. Such initiatives might and indeed, should predicate on feedback obtained from customers as much as possible, although ideas could emanate from whichever source, including expert opinion, of say health personnel, and the shop floor. Considering the interconnectedness of the variety of processes that result eventually in healthcare delivery, the potential complexity of the appropriate approaches to healthcare strategy by corporations is self-evident, not to mention the need for corporations to factor in other elements of the strategy triangle mentioned earlier for example. Also evident is the likely inadequacy of ignoring the need to incorporate new data and information in the processes resulting from the interplay of these processes, in other words, discountenancing the requirement for redundancy to borrow an engineering parlance that could be the lifeline of a seemingly effective strategy, for example. Thus, failure to correspond the firm's strengths with the healthcare needs of its workers on an ongoing basis could negate its efforts to achieve the DHDO, and in the long term compromise its enduring viability, and in particular, not synchronized with its customers' needs and the competitive forces it confronts. In other words, healthcare strategy would increasingly involve more than considerations regarding the workers but would also factor in the other elements of the strategy triangle, at the very least, as the example of the gym-in-the-mall mentioned earlier shows. Thus, firms would have to consider healthcare strategy in the context of their overall business strategy, hence as creating competitive edge at tolerable costs. In other words, firms would increasingly need to differentiate themselves from their competitors, and healthcare strategies could be effective in so doing, in, for example ensuring the recruitment and retention crucial to the sustenance of the human capital on which perhaps survival in an industry precariously depends. Thus, firms are going to use healthcare strategies, singly or in combination with the other elements of the strategy triangle to zero in on key factors of success (KFS) for competitive advantage. This all-inclusive conceptualization of healthcare strategy is going to become increasingly prevalent as businesses seek mileage against competition in novel, even unconventional ways, differently put, 'free-thinking,'or 'out-of-the-box thinking,' which underscores the line-in-loop strategic orientation as itself would be ever more inherent for business success. In other words, just as there would be little if any room for raw intuition as the sole driver of strategy, would it also be unlikely that linear thinking would constitute the panacea strategic-thinking mode, even though elements of both would no doubt feature to a more or less extent in the strategy exercise. Indeed, healthcare strategy, much like any other, would feature not just eclecticism, but also apparent complexity, in its sourcing, which in fact, appropriately conceptualized, would be simplicity belied. In other words, clear thinking on the value of process cycle analysis, and its employment as part of the strategy exercise for example, could only in the end simplify the strategy exercise, the decomposition/exposition exercise that characterize such analyses the potential instruments for revelations that constitute the line-in-loop processes required to move the firm towards achieving its strategic objectives. By determining and starting with the KFS, firms would be able to in turn identify and set in motion, the required analytical pathways from which the required initiatives that would result in the achievement of its goals would emerge, the analyses being ongoing, receptive to the incorporation of new data and information, and to continuous evaluation. The evaluation in particular, would benchmark the performance of the initiatives in ensuring conferment of the competitive edge the firm needs to survive let alone thrive.

The concept of 'line-in-loop' stresses the potential chaos of the strategy process, yet its inherent simplicity. The point is that firms would find it increasingly difficult to disregard interactive iteration in strategy given the forces holding increasing sway in the business world, specifically, the increasing globalization that characterizes the contemporary milieu. Even the big firms would structurally need to 'decompose' to operate more efficiently and effectively in this increasingly fragmented climate, the small businesses with more grassroots affinity, better able to exploit the increasingly superior scope rather than scale economies that the empowerment that networks, social, andothers, increasingly confer. This highlights the need for such small firms to pay more attention to healthcare strategies for the reasons hitherto mentioned among others, for the firms themselves to be competitive. Thus, the issue of workers' health is going to require collaborative efforts at various levels, including governments easing regulations to ensure that these small businesses could afford to offer their workers the sort of healthcare that could make them competitive in an increasingly hyper-competitive global marketplace. Clearly, governments, and indeed, an entire country have high stakes in ensuring that small businesses survive and prosper. In working out their healthcare strategies therefore, companies would be seeking relocations to 'friendly' states and provinces, if not even countries, which is going to play a crucial role in wealth distribution at all levels and in the geo-political/economic world order in the years ahead. Thus, the 'line-in-loop' concept is more inclusive than it appears on the surface to be, as it is reflective of the potential for change that commitment at all levels to the proper conceptualization of the significance of healthcare for our affairs as humans in general could achieve. The significance of that change is in not just raising our living standards, but also in contributing to building a solid economic base for any society, from which would spring 'real power' in the years ahead, as competition for the increasingly scarce resources available to us intensifies, and the futility of enforcement in appropriating the resources become ever more evident. In other words, 'real power' would be the prospects of peoples living healthy, comfortable, peaceful, and meaningful lives, able to realize their potential, and goals, unencumbered by nagging angst on the purpose, meaning, and value, of their very existence. It would become increasingly evident that liberty and the free-market are the crucial political and economic elements required to achieve these goals, hence, which every society would therefore inevitably seek. Considering the role that healthcare plays in realizing the ideals of liberty and free-market operations, it would hardly surprise any then that businesses would increasingly confer on the appropriate strategies to healthcare the necessary priority. Thus, even at the firm's level, the importance of the healthcare strategy to be unforced on the workers is clear. This means that an important aspect of this strategy would be buying-in its end-users, the workers, a critical part of doing so being, involving them with its evolution from the start, in other words seeking their input all the way. Strategy would thus be an increasingly horizontal, bottom-up, rather than a hierarchical, top-down, process, wherein, in the latter case, management just rams down decisions taken at the top on the workers. As noted earlier, firms would increasingly see their workers as customers too, of the health plans and healthcare providers that organize service provision for them, hence recognize that they, the workers have expectations in a customer-centric healthcare delivery milieu. Indeed, underpinning the customer being at the center of the healthcare delivery universe is the liberty to choose, the choice based on rational decision-making, to accomplish which firms would, as strategy, actively engage their efforts. Recognizing that such rational choices could mean more efficient and cost-effective health services utilization, hence reduced healthcare costs, hence spending, firms would doubtless benefit from initiatives that promote such decision-making. As also noted earlier, such efforts by firms would transcend, although should include, information provision, encompassing efforts to encourage workers to actually implement knowledge derived from the information, which clearly coercion would unlikely achieve. In short, entrenching democratic principles in its operations would increasingly be legitimate elements of the healthcare strategy of the firm that intends to succeed. It is clear from our discussion thus far that the idea of the 'line-in-loop' is a comprehensive approach to healthcare and other strategy that would likely increasingly be rendering a firm somewhat furtive ignoring as the benefits of derivable from not so doing would so glaring as to make others those presumed the firm seeks wondering what they are. Besides, it is conjectural what any firm would be trying to achieve not endorsing fundamental principles on which success would increasingly, and one dare says, imperatively, predicate. Indeed, firms would increasingly seek to exploit elements of strategic degrees of freedom to foray into novel healthcare delivery, health and fitness, and other innovations in collaboration with its workers, and based on a thorough understanding of the expectations of its customers, and its industry's competitive climate to outpace competition. The need to outperform their rivals and gain the desired market foothold would be potent drivers of healthcare strategies among firms in the years ahead as they come to understand and accept more readily the seminal role that health and healthcare of their workers could play in their very survival. This would require firms to dig even deeper into the elements of healthcare erstwhile consigned to domains outside of management or the strategy-formulation circle. Businesses would have to cultivate the knack for unconventional thinking in approaching healthcare strategy, and indeed, any other strategy, as our would reshapes our narratives, creating what some might call new ones, but which as our considerations of the 'line-in-loop' concept indicates, is virtually impossible. This is because the lifespan of any 'narrative' predicates on its evolutionary rate, over which the 'narrative' or its progenitors have little if any control, a function of change, whose drivers are inherently not just could be dissimilar, but are also often legion. It is apposite to mention therefore the increasing use of biologics in healthcare, the more common treatment option they are becoming for persons with such disorders as multiple sclerosis, diabetes, cancer, and rheumatoid arthritis, suggestive of this non-linear progression of developments in medicine that would be crucial for firms to be cognizant of in addressing their own strategy issues. With biologics being 25% of global prescriptions currently12 and sales in the US for example, up by 20 percent to $40.3 billion in 200613, biologics would increasingly gain prominence. This is not to mention that of all drug spending, three of the top ten therapeutic classes in sales terms that year were biologics, namely, erythropoietins for treating anemia at number five, antineoplastic monoclonal antibodies for treating cancer at number seven, and insulin sensitizers for treating diabetes at number nine, firms cannot afford to ignore biologics14. Besides their often-larger molecular structures relative to non- biologic prescription drugs, the administration of biologics is often by infusion in a doctor's office, or by self-injection, and they typically need special handling for example refrigeration, patients requiring a lot of support and monitoring, among others. Thus, treatment with biologics could average up to twenty times more than with most of their non-biologic counterparts15. Use of the biologics Enbrel®, Remicade®, or Rituxan® in treating rheumatoid arthritis for example would on average cost US$15,000–$22,450 versus the US$100–$300 that using non-biologics, aspirin, ibuprofen, methotrexate, or prednisone, would, for treating the same condition, on average annually14. Indeed, spending in the US on "specialty pharmaceuticals", to which categories pharmacy benefit managers (PBMs), biologics fall under, increased 16.1 percent, according to Medco, a PBM, and or 21 percent, according to another PBM, Express Scripts, from 2005 to 2006, over double or triple the spending rise on non-specialty drugs14. With biologics providing patients with certain chronic conditions, more favourable long-term outcomes16, we are likely to witness their increasing use in future17, with potentially dire cost implications for businesses, and perhaps implications for access to these medications by their workers. With the costs of biologics billed to be up to US$99 billion by 2010 in the US, or 26 percent of total drug expenditures spending15, firms would need to adopt broader-based approaches to healthcare strategy, which perhaps underlines the establishment recently by the Mexican Billionaire, Carlos Slim Helu, of the Carso Health Institute18. With ever- more worldwide attention on public health as a key player in development, the establishment of an Institute to fund health-related projects and research health priorities in Latin America breaks with the tradition established by, for examples, the Bill and Melinda Gates Foundation and the Global Fund to Fight AIDS,Tuberculosis and Malaria, which fund health programs.

That the Institute Executive President Julio Frenk, Mexico's former health minister and a candidate for head of the World Health Organization (WHO) in 2006, noted that the Institute is a "hybrid organization" that would carry out analyses on major Latin American health issues prior to designing and funding projects to solve them also anchors process cycle analysis in healthcare strategy. It also highlights the trend towards the proactive rather than reactive approach to healthcare issues. Additionally, in relation to these issues, that the Gates Foundation has branched out into global development programs in areas such as agriculture and microfinance emphasizes the multidimensional mindset that contemporary approaches to health issues warrant. The differences in approaches between the Gates Foundation, which does not conduct in-house research, except those concerning what it does, whereas the Carso Institute would, its own researches, is instructive. So is that Gates is investing substantially in biomedical technology development for health, Carso, in Latin American health issues, with a focus on maternal and child health and the Millennium Development Goals (MDGs), and on globalization and noncommunicable diseases and injuries, stressing the 'healthy' eclecticism in approaches to healthcare strategy from which healthcare delivery could only eventually benefit. The premise of action by Carso being the prevalent health problems that Latin America faces, namely chronic diseases, for examples diabetes and cardiovascular diseases, which indeed, are also becoming increasingly prevalent in the developing world in general, as the starting point, would no doubt aid the decomposition/exposition that underlie jurisdictional process cycle analyses. This would in turn, facilitate the emergence of the appropriate healthcare strategies for these problems with local flavour, and perhaps potential for generalizations in some instances. The profound epidemiological transition from communicable to noncommunicable diseases that Latin America has recently been experiencing, noncommunicable diseases (NCDs) and injuries the causes of 69% of deaths and 65% of disability-adjusted life years (DALYs) since the 1990s, and in 2000, 73% of deaths and 65% of DALYs18, underscores the need for attention to these issues, and proactively too. Thus, Carso is simply trailblazing what would, indeed become the concern of businesses large, or small, in the region, and on which in determining their healthcare strategies, they would increasingly focus, in particular as unhealthy lifestyles, and social inequalities are key factors in the changing disease patterns in the region, and indeed, elsewhere. These are issues, in solving which businesses no doubt have key roles to play. Healthcare strategy is likely to feature increasing interests in measures to reduce social inequalities and cultivate healthier lifestyles, in more or less generic and specific terms, depending on the size and resources of the business in question. Thus, it is not going to be possible for all businesses to embark on the initiatives such as those of Gates and Carlos mentioned earlier. However, this does not mean that they cannot contribute to the same causes, in more or less, specific terms with limited focus on their immediate jurisdictions, via initiatives singly, or in collaboration with others, which would help achieve the stated goals. A small firm in addition to for example, encouraging its workers to imbibe the findings in a recent study that the consumption of small amounts of polyphenol-rich dark chocolate as a constituent of a usual diet efficiently reduced elevated blood pressure20, could also help spread the message locally, via for example, paid advertisements in the local media. With the effects of chocolate on blood pressure (Bp) even if small, clinically noteworthy, on a population basis, a 3-mm Hg reduction in systolic BP, potentially cutting the relative risk of stroke mortality by 8 percent, that of coronary artery disease by 5 percent, and of all-cause mortality by 4 percent, such efforts are doubtless worthwhile. In fact, according to the July 29, 2007 issue of Chicago Tribune, an Indiana hospital has set up an in-hospital 'chocolate-wellness café' that offers 'chocolate therapy' 20 an initiative, and others akin to it, which we might start to see established by businesses as part of their healthcare strategy in future. From the cost perspective, that small quantities of commercial cocoa confectionary offer an identical BP-lowering potential as do all-inclusive dietary modifications proven effective in lowering cardiovascular event rate, would interest firms whose dual healthcare strategy objectives of qualitative health services provision and cost containment, consuming the confectionery would serve well. For one is the simplicity of the message of and likelihood of adherence to consuming small amounts of dark chocolate in one's habitual diet versus to complex behavioural changes and extensive counselling sessions inherent in some traditional behavioural modification approaches to lowering blood pressure in individuals with above-optimal blood pressure. Besides, these latter approaches are also clearly likely to be costlier. These issues also point to the important role the 'line-in-loop' approach to healthcare strategy would increasingly play regardless of the size of the business. The essential element of this approach being the adoption of a flexible, interactive iteration of processes involved in determining initiatives and acting upon them that would enable the firm achieve its DHDO, is likely to gain further currency, given its potential to benefit the firm, regarding its bottom line, but in the initiatives constituting a veritable social leverage. This, considering the fragmentation in the business milieu that globalization would increasingly engender, would bring the values of such social advantage in boosting a firm's local standing, increasing its customer base, and securing the loyalty of these customers, squarely to the fore. In other words, and as earlier noted, part of the success-driving, healthcare strategy of the future, would predicate on its differentiation capacity in beating competition. This would be hardly achievable by the firm sticking to a narrow, inflexible 'strategic planning' mindset, with its formulate-then-implement underpinning, with little if any room for incorporating novel ideas and information in iterative loops into the strategy process to modify, and improve it. Whereas, novelty rooted in eclecticism, the curious admixture of rationality, intuition, and creativity, for examples, are surely the ingredients of the motion of great companies that create markets as opposed to even good ones that merely meet market needs. Healthcare strategy seems likely poised to play a significant role in making the difference between the two in the years ahead, not to mention between them and those others whose very survival would become increasingly precarious the longer they tarry adopting the strategic approaches best suited to the new economic dispensation.

References:

1. Zook C. Recognize the Power of Repeatability in the Core. Harvard Business Online. Available at: http://conversationstarter.hbsp.com/2007/07/recognize_the_power_of_repeata

.html Accessed on July 29, 2007

2. Sull DN. Closing the Gap Between Strategy and Execution. MITSloan Management Review. Reprint 48412; summer 2007, Vol. 48, No. 4, pp. 30-38 Available at: http://sloanreview.mit.edu/smr/issue/2007/summer/12/

3. Christakis NA, Fowler JH. The spread of obesity in a large social network over 32 years. N Engl J Med 2007; 357:370-9.

4. Frayling TM, Timpson NJ, Weedon MN, et al. A common variant in the FTO gene is associated with body mass index and predisposes to childhood and adult obesity. Science 2007; 316:889-94.

5. Barabasi A. Network Medicine-From Obesity to the "Diseaseome". N Engl J Med 2007; 357:404

6. Barabási A-L, Oltvai ZN. Network biology: understanding the cell's functional organization. Nat Rev Genet 2004; 5:101-15

7. Available at:

http://www.msnbc.msn.com/id/20036086/wid/11915773?GT1=10212&print=1

&displaymode=1098 Accessed on July 30, 2007

8. Tirosh, A. The New England Journal of Medicine, Oct. 6, 2005, vol 353: pp 1454- 1462.

9. Simon J, Pilling S, Burbeck R, Goldberg D. Treatment options in moderate and severe depression: decision analysis supporting a clinical guideline. Br. J. Psychiatry, Dec 2006; 189: 494 - 501.

10. Kuhn, T.S. "The Function of Dogma in Scientific Research". Pp. 347-69 in A. C. Crombie (ed.) Scientific Change (Symposium on the History of Science, University of Oxford, 9-15 July 1961). New York and London: Basic Books and Heinemann, 1963.

11. Kuhn, T.S. The Structure of Scientific Revolutions. Chicago: University of Chicago Press, 1962. ISBN 0-226-45808-3

12. "The Global Biotech Report 2006," Visiongain, Sept 2006.

13. IMS Health, Press Release, March 8, 2007.

14. Rucker N Lee. Biologics in Perspective: Expanded Clinical Options amid Greater Cost Scrutiny. AARP Public Policy Institute Publication. June 2007

15. Express Scripts, "Biotech Drug Spending Increases 21 Percent Even as Growth in Rx Expenditure Slows", Press Release, April 25, 2007.

16. Diaz-Borjon A, Weyand CM, Goronzy JJ. "Treatment of Chronic

Inflammatory Diseases with Biologic Agents: Opportunities and Risks for the Elderly," Experimental Gerontology 41(12) (Dec. 2006): 1250–55.

17. Gabriel SE, Coyle D, Moreland LW, "A Clinical and Economic Review of Disease-Modifying Antirheumatic Drugs", Pharmacoeconomics 19(7) (2001): 715–28.

18. Available at: http://www.who.int/bulletin/volumes/85/8/07-

010807/en/index.html Accessed on August 3, 2007

19. Available at: http://enews.ama-assn.org/t/27764/305999/167/0/ Accessed on August 3, 2007

20. Available at: http://enews.ama-assn.org/t/27764/305999/168/0/ Accessed on August 3, 2007

Employer-Sponsored Health Insurance and Healthcare Quality

The debate on healthcare financing rages, fiercer in particular in the US lately preparatory it appears to the 2008 presidential elections. Proponents of universal coverage refer to the large numbers of Americans lacking health insurance, disparities in accessibility even among those that do due to, among other reasons, the vagaries of employer-sponsored insurance. About 160 million Americans, two thirds of the country's nonelderly population had employer-sponsored healthcare coverage in 2004[1]. Yet, despite that there was no significant increase in the percentage of uninsured individuals in the country in 2004, fewer workers and their families now have employment-based health benefits, 64.4 percent in 1994 versus 62.4 percent in 2004, for example, although coverage expanded between 1994 and 2000 to surpass the growth in public health programs. In fact, there has been a steady increase in the growth of public-sector health coverage, which rose to 17.5 percent of the nonelderly population in 2004, Medicaid, and the State Children's Health Insurance Program(SCHIP) enrolment also increasing by 1.8 million in the same year, providing coverage for 13.4 percent of the nonelderly population, versus 10.5 percent in 1999[1]. Thus, public healthcare coverage in the country is increasing as employer-based health coverage declines. Given the yearly drop in health insurance coverage in the country except for two years since 1994, when 36.5 million nonelderly individuals were uninsured, the uninsured population in 2004, 45.5 million[1], it is clear that either the increase in public health coverage is not enough, or the decline in employer-sponsored insurance is too much. These figures could thus strengthen the positions by purveyors of both possibilities, of the former for calls for universal healthcare coverage, and of the latter for advocating promoting rather than destroying employer-based insurance, on which so many Americans rely for their health services provision. Yet, others would remind us promptly that we are still here simply examining figures relating to access to healthcare, and not necessarily indicative of the quality of service provision. Interestingly, the percentage of health coverage individuals bought on their own in 2004 remained relatively unchanged at about 6.5% since 1994. This, if we were to consider price a key driver of such purchases, suggests that other factors, perhaps outside the control of employers, drive coverage costs up, or compromise in other ways, the ability of these employers to provide their workers with healthcare coverage without risking going out of business. The destabilizing, some would argue, unintended consequences of the Employee Retirement Income Security Act (ERISA) enacted in 1974, the law actually aimed at protecting employees against the malpractices of those investing their pension funds and other benefits, is instructive in this regard. This is so, in not only that in enabling some major employers to extract from the health insurance risk pool their healthy and wealthier workers, which spiked premiums, essentially edging out smaller employers, it contributed to the fall in the numbers of workers covered[2], but also, it soon became the albatross of states pursuing universal health coverage objectives. In the latter instance, by exempting firms that provided their workers healthcare coverage from state regulation of this coverage, it enabled firms to dodge state mandates to cover certain services with the potential to increase costs, and because state approval was not required, to develop novel, some would insist, cost-curtailing, coverage packages[2]. Thus, the law favoured some employers, did not, others, compromised free-market operations in the insurance industry, with its fallout, a decline in the number of workers on employer-sponsored health insurance, but it also compromised the ability of states to enhance health services accessibility and quality, all no doubt, not intended goals of the legislation. Nor probably were they, the nature and scope of the 'horror' the 1990 ruling by the Financial Accounting Standards Board (FASB), the Financial Accounting Statement No. 106 (FAS 106), mandating with effect from 1992[3], companies covering retired employees' health care expenses to include future retiree health benefit liabilities on their financial statements[4,5], visited on these companies. FAS 106 reduced companies' assets essentially[5], compromising their share prices, impelling containment, with resultant disinterest by companies in health services coverage for their workers. Incidentally, with a recent similar ruling suggestive of the public sector facing similar accounting standards and similar cost pressures, it is plausible that the effects on access to care would be unlikely positive, calling the benefits of 'mandating' universal coverage into question. Indeed, in an article titled 'Whence And Whither Health Insurance? A Revisionist History' published in the journal Health Affairs in 2005, Moran[2] in which he noted that policymakers have, since post-WWII, aimed to expand both public and private insurance coverage, simultaneously struggling with the costs implications of the resultant insurance-financing mechanisms, advanced what some would deem a startling position. He contended that the US had reached the limits to insurance expansion and that public and private plan sponsors would thenceforth 'thin out' what coverage they offer on an ongoing basis, offering 'direct service delivery' as an option for mitigating access concerns. Indeed, as with Moran, and as business-as-usual, 'health policy as ideological struggle' as it might sound, the crucial point is the need to appreciate and acknowledge the paradigmatic shift underpinning the redundancy of the 'regulatory cost-control v. market-oriented strategies' model of conceptualizing healthcare financing in not just the US, but elsewhere, impelled by change. In other words, by developments in medicine, and technology, for examples, and indeed, in the global economy, and which would continue, being inherent in change, which itself is inevitable. This presumably allows atonement for our past mistakes, but does it excuse us from making new ones, in particular stuck in a dated mindset, a simplistic dichotomization of vital issues with the potential to compromise us, amplifying the pervasive existential angst with whose paradox we constantly struggle to resolve? Still in the US, is it not instructive that even with veto-proof Democratic majorities in both Houses of Congress, President Jimmy Carter's proposed legislation to curtail increasing hospital costs to minimize the eventual cost of universal insurance coverage was stuck in a regulation/competition debate in the Ninety-fifth and Ninety-sixth Congresses[2]? Or not, that all nine Republican presidential candidates, on Sunday August 05, 2007 during a debate held on the campus of Drake University in Des Moines, Iowa, and moderated by ABC's 'This Week' host George Stephanopoulos, opposed a bill that the Senate recently passed that would reauthorize and expand SCHIP, and which President Bush has threatened to veto[6]? What should one make of the findings of a study by the Massachusetts Medical Society released on July 24 2007 that 49% of internists in the state are not accepting new patients, regarding the success or otherwise of its universal coverage plans[7]? In fact, the top three teaching hospitals in Boston indicate that 95% of their 270 doctors in general practice no longer enroll patients[7], and the medical society that the state's residents able to get an appointment with their primary care doctor have to wait on the average for over seven weeks. It is thus, unlikely unreasonable to wonder with the primary care system already under such strain, how doctors in the state would accommodate an added half-million patients in quest of checkups and other routine healthcare. The point is there is shortage of primary care doctors, including internists, family physicians, and paediatricians, across the US. According to the Centre for Studying Health System Change in Washington, the numbers of these doctors fell 6% relative to the general population from 2001 to 2005, and that just 25% of third-year internal medicine residents are opting to practice primary care in 2005, versus 54% in 19987. Across the country, 13% of family medicine positions remain vacant at federally financed health centres, a 2006 JAMA study noted 7. The so-called 'numerus clausus' policies, cost-containment measures many countries implemented during the 1980s and 1990s that reduced the number of new doctors through limiting medical school intakes, apart, and despite the increase between 1990 and 2005 in the ratio of practicing doctors per 1000 population, among almost all Organization for Economic Cooperation and Development (OECD) countries, is telling8. This is more so given that in most of these countries, according to the OECD Health Data 2007, the increasing numbers of specialists, up nearly 50% between 1990 and 2005, versus the 20% increase in general practitioners (GPs), seem to be driving this growth8, income the real driver. Also according to these data, from 1990 to 2005, there was a fall in the annual number of medical students graduating in France, Germany, Italy, Japan Spain, and Switzerland. It noted the prospects if training efforts did not improve notably, of reliance by these countries rely increasingly on foreign-trained doctors as 'baby-boomer' doctors retire. It is hardly debatable that fewer numbers of doctors per capita could cause longer waiting times for both outpatient and inpatient services, or that countries would not need to focus more on pressing issues such as the shortage of professionals, including recruitment and retention, tied invariably with methods of recompense, rather than on ideological power play. On another, yet related dimension the question of what the quality of health services has to do, with considerations of access to healthcare to many people, would be likely moot, as would whether this would not put any health system, privately or publicly financed under some pressure, costs for example, or another. Indeed, it is conceivable to argue thereon from the perspective of the degree of costs pressure for example that either health-financing model would be on, to justify not only the dichotomy, but also the supremacy, hence the ascendancy of one or the other of its elements, and still be missing the point. Yet, the importance of, and indeed, the urgency for us, not to miss this crucial point, one cannot gainsay. What is more, in many countries, including the US, Canada, and the UK, the two principal health-financing systems already operate in tandem and indeed, the ratio in perpetual flux as the graph below of public share of healthcare expenditures among OECD countries shows.

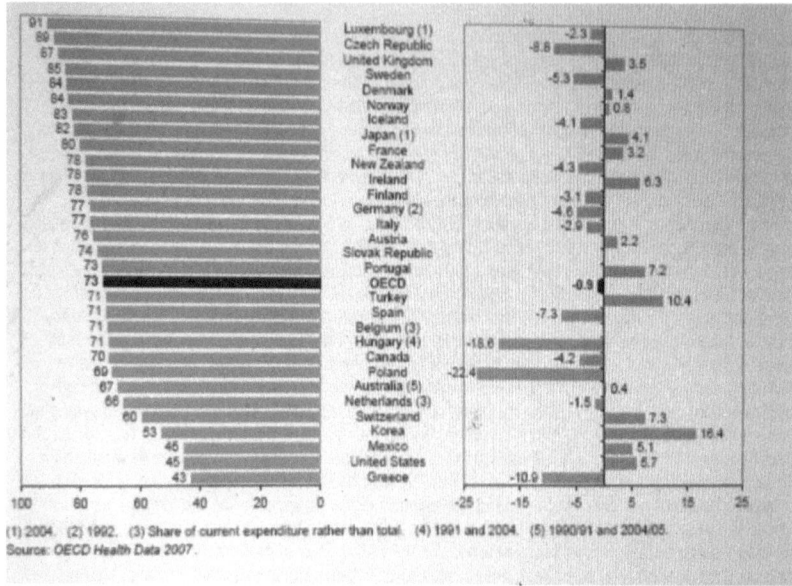

(1) 2004. (2) 1992. (3) Share of current expenditure rather than total. (4) 1991 and 2004. (5) 1990/91 and 2004/05.
Source: OECD Health Data 2007.

Thus, besides the need for cautious management and planning of the medical workforce in keeping with a country's present and future health care needs, never mind its seeming stealth among issues bogging down health systems across the globe, countries would need to take other measures to leash soaring healthcare costs, the key driver of health sector reforms (HSF). Thus, they might have to increase taxes or social security quotas, slash spending in other areas, or out-of-pocket health expenses might increase if, as is currently the case with many countries, health spending kept outpacing economic growth. Among OECD countries for example, per capita health spending rose by over 80% in real terms between 1990 and 2005, on average outpacing the 37% growth in GDP per capita8. From an average among OECD countries of just 5% of GDP in 1970, health spending was 7% by 1990, and is 9% at present. One in four OECD countries now spends more than 10% of its income on health. With a 15.3% share in 2005, the United States leads by a wide margin, followed by Switzerland (11.6%), France (11.1%), and Germany (10.7%). Yet, they would also need to address other issues besides costs, for example, service efficiency, and quality, which is not to say, that they do not impinge on costs, or vice versa. Indeed, they would need to reorient toward achieving what we would call the dual healthcare delivery objectives (DHDO), essentially aiming for accessible and qualitative health services provision simultaneously reducing healthcare costs, hence expenditures, regardless of whether they opt for 'socialized medicine' or 'free-market medicine' or whatever taxonomic entity it is. Crucially therefore, what has employer-based health insurance got to do with achieving these objectives, in particular if we were thinking it would facilitate their realization, and given also that the country in question operated or opted for publicly funded healthcare delivery model? That reform efforts could contain soaring healthcare costs is sufficient reason to engage in these efforts as an ever-increasing healthcare costs is simply unsustainable in no country. However, for these reforms to succeed, countries need to recognize and address the many underlying pressures contributing to healthcare spending increase, for example, demographic changes, aging in developed countries to be more specific, which would not only increase health spending, but along with increasing expenditures on pensions, would be a potent pressure point for these economies. In these countries therefore, the need to seek ways to reduce public healthcare spending and reform pensions policies is going to be an urgent priority in the near future, if not already so as even expecting their essentially diminishing working-age population to maintain retirees would become unrealistic sooner than later, and a potential source of social tension. A recent OECD Economics Department working paper 149 that reviewed trends in health-care expenditure and evaluated the main forces underlying health-spending increases since 1960, among others noted that top-down budget controls seemed to have helped reduce healthcare spending growth, although emphasized microeconomic reforms along with this approach to be sustainable8. Thus, the countries it seems must reform their health services or face some potentially dire consequences, and as we would argue here, businesses have a key role to play in this exercise. The elements of health sector reform (HSR) are varied, including increased 'empowerment' through enhanced healthcare consumer choice and provider autonomy9. However, in general, reforms aim for, among three main goals, equitable service provision, which guarantees access, based on need and not income, and shelters individuals the financial costs of being ill, payment for which, as private or social insurance, income transfers or public, supply, ought to be income-not risk-related9. As mentioned earlier, the OECD study noted the importance of improvements in micro-efficiency and effectiveness in driving down healthcare costs, and specifically recommended incentives to healthcare providers. In the U.S., a bipartisan bill in the Senate, the Wired for Health Care Quality Act, includes $278 million in matching grants to assist doctors purchase healthcare information technology clearly is in this direction10, as should similar efforts by the private sector. Indeed, the report observed that policy developments in a few key OECD countries indicate that a system 'where funders/insurers act as purchasers, contracting with competing health-care providers, is a promising model for reform.9 This observation is pertinent vis-à-vis the intricacies of the inherent principal-agent transactions. This is so in particular in light for example, of reports that at the 2006 American Medical Association (AMA) Annual Meeting, delegates adopted policy that said that public and private payers should not require physicians to use electronic medical records (EMRs10.) Even given that some studies have called into question the ability of the technologies to improve healthcare delivery quality10, others have given them accolades in this regard. A systematic review of 257 studies for example, published in the May 16 2006 issue of the journal, The Annals of Internal Medicine, found that many doctors using EMRs 'increased their adherence to care guidelines, committed fewer medication errors, and monitored patients more closely10.' The policy therefore points to the difficulties that might arise in the actualizing efforts such as the OECD recommendation clearly aims to do, to improve the quality of health services' and reduce costs, but which we contend businesses could achieve via employer-sponsored health insurance, and which in fact is in their best interests so to do. This would involve a completely new way by businesses of viewing their involvement in health services provision, whose mechanics would in full glow, manifest in what might seem to be dramatic supply and demand ends modifications in the interplay of market forces, to which such policies as that of the AMA mentioned above would naturally defer. We would see complementary initiatives from government such as for example, in the US legislations such asthe Health Professions Education Act of 1963 (P.L. 88-204), which signalled a serious commitment to the expansion of the professional service supply. We would not see wanton infrastructure development, or any other incredulous supply side initiative not supported by developments in the prevailing, hence inherently, fluid zeitgeist, the appropriate responses to which we would rationally, seek. Is it any wonder that public service mechanisms seem to lack so much credence, as we evidently suggest, when even a quite reasonable commitment to the administrative backbone of health sector reform (HSR), by many countries, including developed countries, would hardly materialize? Never mind, that commitment to this New Public Management (NPM), essentially the public service operating in a private enterprise paradigm, and as Kaul (1997)11 noted, is government moving from 'a concern to do, towards a concern to ensure that things are done,' which clearly would, NPM aims, enhance its efficiency, and cost-effectiveness. This would seem, already to be building the case for the superior efficiency of private sector operations over those of the public sector, and indirectly of that of market forces driving health services than central planning, but the issues are more fundamental, and implicitly actually simpler, rather than more complex, conceptualized appropriately. In fact, rather than prescribe heavy supply and demand constraints does, as some would expect, and which the present, and indeed, historical, picture, to a certain extent of the involvement of businesses in healthcare provision would suggest, the efforts would, at the very least, rather aim to optimize resources at reasonable costs. Given the sort of appreciation by businesses of their role and its significance in this regard, achieving these goals is certainly doable, and indeed, desirable. Given for example, the increasing globalization that compels an appreciation of the need for competitiveness amongst businesses wherever they are more than ever before, are the prospects of these businesses carrying on business as usual likelier than more focus on such resource optimization, including in their healthcare strategies? In a testimony to the House Small Business Committee Hearing on 'U.S. Trade Policy and Small Business' on June 13, 200712, Daniel Griswold, Director, Centre for Trade Policy Studies, Cato Institute emphasized the country's earnings via the export of goods and services and from foreign investments abroad reached a record 15.6 percent of gross domestic product (GDP). He also noted that spending on imported goods and services and payments on investments, reached a record 22.2 percent of GDP, figures that attest to the immense growth opportunities for US small businesses in the global markets. Further, he stressed the benefits that U.S. small businesses have derived from exporters into an ever-increasing global market, including China, and that in 2006, U.S. exports of goods to other countries reached $1 trillion for the very first time, exports of services, also a record $422 billion. These opportunities indeed, also abound for small businesses in other countries, but whether these businesses, or the circumstances under which they operate would allow them to exploit the opportunities, is another matter. Could small businesses, and indeed, large ones, afford to go under given these potential prospects, and should any economy allow them to? Is it not therefore clear, that indeed, both the public and private sectors should be keenly aware of the stakes and ensure that health services provision is cost-effective and efficient to ensure the creation and continuity of the enabling milieu for businesses and indeed, the economy to thrive? Considering, the legendary bureaucracies that bog down public sector operations, what role should the private sector have in ensuring the efficient and cost-effective, delivery of health services to their workers, and their dependants, in indirectly to the rest of the populace? Should it not consider this role indeed a responsibility, for its own sake, and for the sake of the economy in which it operates?

The point in fact is, and as deemed, a second of three key goals of HSR, micro-economic efficiency, the maximization and at minimal costs of care quality and consumer satisfaction, is indispensable to the realization of these healthcare delivery objectives be it in the private or public health sector. Thus, the institution of appropriate organizational structures and technologies such as healthcare information and communication technologies (healthcare ICT) to enhance resource optimization, cognizance of the deleterious effects on the workforce of diseases, and in tandem with attention to developments in medical practice would contribute to finding, implementing, and evaluating the most efficient and cost-effective ways to boost health 'outcomes.' This would ensure not only the establishment getting stuck in flawed healthcare strategies, but also that health spending is under control, and in the case of government, not compromising its ability to deliver other services, and of companies, if not even threatening their very survival. The stakes are clearly high and the prospects of firms designing their healthcare strategies to ensure that they, the firms, do not go under, literally, underscores the point about the value of employer-sponsored health insurance in improving healthcare quality. Even regarding macroeconomic cost control, the third key HSR goal, whose underlying thrust is for the health sector using an apposite percentage of GDP, employer-sponsored health insurance appropriately envisioned and implemented could help obviate market failure resulting in surplus health services supply or demand, with spending curtailed just as many governments now do, struggling to curtail 'runaway' health spending. Given the potential for soaring health expenditures to drive companies aground, employer-sponsored health insurance would likely be cognizant of and prevent to major features of the health market that could result in excess services provision namely, information asymmetry and moral hazard. By preferring for example to purchase services from providers that have mechanisms in place to rectify information asymmetry, for example, that provide information on services/products pricing, companies via employer-sponsored health insurance would be averting or mitigating this aspect of market failure. In other words, companies would be more inclined to seek to provide their workers with the necessary information for rational decision making regarding matters of health, knowing this would facilitate the achievement of the DHDO. Ordinarily, this should also be the case in the public sector, but with choices of providers for example, limited, and given the remuneration structures of providers, typically centralized, fee-for-service (FFS), for example, and services being free, the potential for overuse/ abuse of services are real, as are the difficulties preventing such practices. This results in demand-side moral hazard as consumers do not pay or pay minimally for the services, but also supply-side moral hazard as a third party pays for the services, which suppliers oversupply. Furthermore, with most patients lacking vital information to make rational choices, which leaves them little if any choices than to entrust, more or less, treatment decisions to doctors and other healthcare providers, also the services suppliers, the potential for a conflict of interest in the principal/ agent dyadic is rife, compromising service quality, increasing overall costs of the transactions involved. Given the modus operandi in the private sector relative to the public sector, and in particular, the bureaucratic machinery and the non-for-profit orientation of the latter, in the main, that the private sector, via employer-sponsored health insurance would indeed, seek to and likely achieve improvement in the access to, and quality of health services delivery seems quite probable. Indeed, in the US for example, many would contend that employer-sponsored health insurance has been doing just that, providing the vital keystone of an insurance system by engendering employment-based risk pools, wherein healthy, low-risk members subsidize the healthcare costs of ill, high-risk ones, affordably, albeit buoyed by liberal federal tax subsidies. There is no doubt that in countries such as the US where businesses fund healthcare substantially, to assume that its ramifications for healthcare efficiency, cost-effectiveness, and quality could be immense is hardly questionable, as is that of the intention and willingness to sponsor, and engage in health reform being crucial to the overall effective operations of the entire health system. Companies could be key determinants of the evolution of novel health insurance products and services that would ensure service quality improvement as they modulate market operations wherein private insurers compete for employers' business. This is evident in the string of new models of healthcare coverage, including the early 1990s' managed care reforms, and more recently pay-for-performance (P4P), health savings accounts (HSA), disease-management approaches, tiered-payments model, and consumer-directed health plans, among others, some of these models, adopted by other countries, for example P4P for GPs in England. This attests to interests in innovative approaches to healthcare spawned by employer-sponsored insurance, even in other countries, and its potential to improve healthcare delivery quality, among others. Wholesale public sector cost control measures, for example, the overt regulatory restraints on allowable high-end hospital revenue growth that the Carter administration in the US proposed for limiting demand and that was antecedent to efforts a decade or two later to abolish retrospective cost reimbursement of hospitals preferentially to managed pricing arrangements determined upfront, worked 2. Perhaps, administered price regimes worked, we should say, only to a certain extent, and resulted for example, in a record fall in Medicare expenditures in the late 1990s, buoyed by the 1997 Balanced Budget Act (BBA). Yet, price control alone is inadequate to rein in summative costs successfully, and indeed, tend to encourage an increase by providers in service volume to counterbalance the resultant income deficits as critics of FFS would readily contend. In short, the public sector is unlikely to curtail soaring healthcare costs given the cost management mechanisms it has, which further highlights the need to engage the private sector, via the promotion of unfettered market operations such as the employer-sponsored health insurance model creates, in this exercise. Regarding this though, skeptics would ballyhoo the adverse effects on the workers' healthcare risk pool of 1974's Employee Retirement Income Security Act (ERISA) (P.L. 93-406) because, besides its exemption from state regulation, of its offering a regulatory scaffold amiable to conversion of employer-sponsored plans to less costly, self-funded types, rather than paying premiums2. Even smaller firms exploited such self-funded products as the minimum premium plans, the overall result, massive workers' exodus from the insured pool, a hike in the risk profile of the small group and individual insurance markets, hence increased premiums, and compromised coverage. As not even the resulting enactment of the 'corrective' Health Insurance Portability and Accountability Act (HIPAA) of 1996 (PL. 104-191), could reverse the cumulative financial effect of this exodus, cautionary reminders of these pitfalls of what some would regard as the exuberant zeal of the private sector to control costs are quite in order. This is so, even as the reforms of managed care have also highlighted the limits of market tolerability for these control measures2. Yet, we cannot discountenance the findings of a recent study published in the journal Health Affairs that the rates in 2004, charged to many uninsured and other 'self- pay' patients. The rates, for these patients who they or their insurer does not have a contract with the hospital, and of whom the forty-five million uninsured Americans represent the majority, for hospital services were frequently 2.5 times what most health insurers actually paid. They were also often over thrice the hospital's Medicare-allowable costs13. This growing chasm between rates charged to self-pay patients and to other payers has the potential to exclude some, particularly the uninsured from access to hospital care. Besides the three specific policy options that the author suggested in addressing this problems, namely, a voluntary effort by hospitals in particular regarding pricing transparency, litigation, and legislation, the problem might indicate changing market preferences hence would it be best to allow market forces to rectify it? Could this, sustained, not reverse the tendency towards consumers exiting the healthcare risk pool, lowering premiums, expanding coverage? Therefore, even if there were also concerns in certain quarters regarding the tension between compensation costs from the employers' perspective, and the net income accruing, from the workers' perspective in any consideration of costs control by employers, vis-à-vis negotiations with employees, could the operations of market forces not assuage them? This is besides that the question remains in whose interests for example, it is workers essentially being able to tailor their own benefits with novel models such as consumer-directed health plans, opting as the young and healthy in the main seem wont to do, for other forms of compensation and more cost-effective coverage, thus slashing demand for services.

In other words, companies would have to wager over spending less, versus creating an increasing pool of the uninsured, in the main, the young, and healthy, hence who skew the risk pool, making health insurance even costlier. Yet, firms do not have to insist on more cost sharing, or some would argue less coverage, and increased stress on catastrophic benefits. Indeed, it is not in their best interests for able-bodied young persons to be uninsured, or for that matter, the many retirees and those near retirement many employers now no longer offer coverage. That in many developed countries, provision would increasingly be necessary for workers to work past current retirement age if they wished, given the constriction in the labor force that an increasingly aging population in these countries would create, underscores the point on the one hand. It also does that because young people, who would probably still, constitute the majority of the labor force, could also become ill, need, and use significant healthcare resources, on the other, it is important to address their healthcare coverage issues. Many young adults frequently eat fast food, for example, and are far likelier to gain weight and develop type 2 diabetes than those who do not , and with obesity, annually the cause of about 300,000 deaths, and about $100 billion in medical expenditures, it is difficult to ignore the potential contributions to these statistics made by young adults14. Indeed, the average spending per person among young adults aged 18-24 years in the US in 2004 was $1,282, roughly the same as for children, although significantly less than for persons aged over 64 years, for example, who spent per person in the same year, $8,647 15. In the US, young adults (ages 19 to 29) constitute one of the largest segments of the uninsured, 13.3 million lacking coverage in 200516. Yet, lack of health insurance compromises access to the health system by this critical group, creates obstacles to care when required, and exposes them and their families to risks for high out- of-pocket costs during a serious illness or injury, which funds many probably lack16. Additionally in the US, 14 percent of adults ages 18 to 29 are obese, obesity increasing in the 1990s by 70 percent among young adults, the fastest rate of increase among all adults17, 18, which underscores the point made earlier about obesity and type 2 diabetes. Furthermore, there are 3.5 million pregnancies every year among the 21 million women ages 19 to 29, and a third of all HIV diagnoses occur among young adults13. Besides, could companies afford to compromise their ability to compete on the global market creating unhealthy workforce, with compromised productivity? Indeed, that there is little doubt about the direction of healthcare coverage being increasingly unsustainable for the public sector to continue to expand, in cost terms, at least, with the private sector likely to play an increasing role in all countries, regardless of their health financing model buttresses the point about health coverage for young people being a priority. This means the need to explore the prospects and challenges of collaboration between the public and private sectors, in particular for the public sector to provide coverage to those that the private sector could not, for whatever reasons. The increased involvement of the private sector in health insurance is thus, likely to be a process that would be essentially imperative, as would the need for it to ensure that it does so most efficiently and cost-effectively. This it would do, bearing in mind not only the ramifications for itself, and the employees, but also for the entirety of the economy of the country in question. Some have suggested that the direct care delivery system, along the Veterans Administration (VA) medical model would increasingly emerge in the US in lieu of more public insurance making up for the flaws (in particular, the shrinking coverage towards catastrophic-based coverage) of private insurance, in the direction of which latter the motion of health services in the country essentially heads2. There is no doubt about the tension inherent in the key-player dynamics that would emerge in a regime of soaring healthcare costs, contentious demographic mix, the centrality of immigration in a globalized economy literally coming to roost, and the political conundrum resultant. Yet, attention to the underlying fundamental dynamics would offer the best hope of the design of the appropriate policies moving forward. In other words, an acknowledgement of the fact of the need to pursue the dual healthcare delivery objective (DHDO) for example, would highlight the redundancy of any dichotomy of health financing schemes. It would also underline the ascendancy of the operations of market forces being best suited to modulate the interplay of the variables inherent in the evolution of any health system. The real issue then would be seeking the most appropriate approaches to the collaborative efforts on which the success of efforts to realize the DHDO would crucially hinge. In other words, even the firms would realize the futility in the unregulated motion toward the catastrophic-mode approach to employer -sponsored health insurance, emphasizing instead, the appropriate strategies to ensuring the health and wellbeing of its workforce, for via disease prevention, and health promotion, among others. Since it would be in their best interests to have a labor force capable of the productivity levels that would ensure that the companies are able to compete favourably at home and abroad, firms would be more proactive in these domains of healthcare than waiting for disease to occur and becoming embroiled in the techno-medico-legal complexity of disease management. The increasing emphasis on disease prevention and health promotion sustained would reduce focus on coverage for disease management, overhauling in the long-term, the entire concept of health insurance, and the dynamics of the health insurance industry, vis-à-vis the health and other industries involved in the supply/ demand operations of healthcare delivery. Progress in technology would reorient along these lines, as the demand for costly, 'disease management' technologies, with nonetheless incremental health and financial benefits of the sorts that hitherto bogged down the health system in many countries with soaring costs, would dim. Firms would in fact, as opposed to increasingly reducing coverage extent, actually sponsor research into for example, genome studies, which could reveal novel approaches to preempting diseases, by recognizing their presence even before they manifest. Indeed, such research might then be able to do something to reengineer the genes, or the environment in which the individual operates, to forestall the manifestation of the disease, which in totality would ensure the availability of the crucial healthy-workforce, that businesses need to survive in an increasingly competitive, global economy, in particular in economies wherein it is essentially, dwindling. There is no doubt about the need to provide health coverage for all, including those not working. Indeed, firms would also need to factor into their healthcare strategies, the potential effects on their workers' productivity, and indeed, health and wallet, of family members lacking healthcare coverage. That the relative proportion of the population uninsured in the US despite its enormous health expenditures continues to increase underscores the urgency of finding solutions to the issues involved, including that of businesses becoming involved in so doing. Recent data as the chart below shows, on health insurance from the US National Health Interview Survey20 show slight increases in uninsured adults, with 14.8 percent of Americans, or 43.6 million in 2006 currently without health insurance, 19.8 percent among working-age adults (those ages 18-64), 19.8%, an increase in the percent uninsured from 18.9% in 2005. About 9.3% of children under the age of 18 lacked coverage, a non-significant increase in the uninsured from 8.9% in 2005. Incidentally, by definition, someone is uninsured if he or she did not have any private health insurance, Medicare, Medicaid, State Children's Health Insurance Program (SCHIP), state-sponsored or other government-sponsored health plan, or military plan. A person is also uninsured if he or she had only Indian Health Service coverage or had only a private plan that paid for one type of service such as the taxpayer than otherwise. These latter issues highlight the potential for the private sector to participate in this exercise, and the importance of collaborating with the public sector, in reducing the impact of moral hazard and adverse selection. They also stress the redundancy of the dichotomy of health financing as the ultimate goal of either universal coverage or market-based health insurance is the provision of qualitative and accessible health services, cost-effectively and efficiently, which would require major adjustments in both models to address moral hazard and adverse selection, among other issues. Even if universal coverage implies there would be no adverse selection as there are no differential premium rates, and everyone has coverage, there is still 'virtual' information asymmetry, the entire system would suffer because of the reckless behaviour of some, for example, smokers, the public insurer meanwhile unable to act even knowing the smokers. The increased costs thereof would pass on in the form of higher taxes, to keep service delivery going as usual, or service shrinkage, to slash costs and avoid tax hikes. Thus, the publicly funded health system would still need to take measures such as firms would to obviate these problems. In other words, it is clear the potential problems that

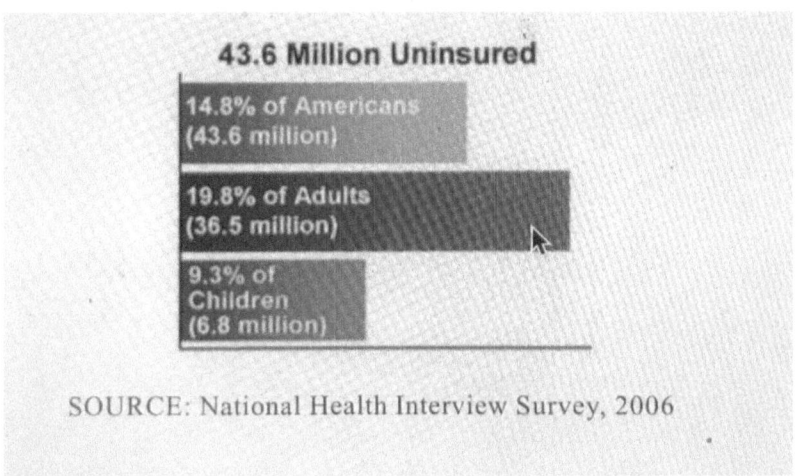

universal coverage pose, which make the potential for its 'perpetual' expansion at once real, and unsustainable, hence essentially unrealistic. It also brings the need for market forces being operational as a crucial approach to ensuring widespread health services delivery squarely to the fore. Indeed, besides the inherent 'private sector' operational practices that tend toward efficiency and cost-effectiveness potentially rubbing off literally via businesses' healthcare strategies, on the firms they also would on the entire healthcare system. Thus, not only would these practices ensure that the firms realize the DHDO, the services delivered by 'public' insurance, would need to operate on similar 'efficiency' principles to survive. In other words, every public health hospital would need to justify its existence sooner than later, which would no doubt be increasingly difficult with the standards of services provision improved among providers to firms, due to certain measures these firms took. It would be increasingly difficult because of the potential loss of patronage by the public health system, if not as efficient, as market forces, would have made access to private health services more affordable. In effect, in improving the efficiency of healthcare services in its domain, employer-sponsored health insurance would also do the same in others, indeed, in the entire health system.

References:

1. Fronstin P. Sources of health insurance and characteristics of the uninsured: analysis of the March 2005 current population survey. Issue brief. No. 287. Washington, D.C.: Employee Benefits Research Institute, 2005.
Available at http://www.ebri.org/pdf/briefspdf/EBRI_IB_11-20051.pdf. Accessed on August 6, 2007.

2. Moran DW. Whence and whither health insurance? A revisionist history. Health Aff (Millwood) 2005; 24:1415-25

3. Blumenthal D. Employer-Sponsored Health Insurance in the United States: Origins and Implications. N Engl J Med 355:82, July 6, 2006 Health Policy Report

4. Igelhart JK. Changing health insurance trends. N Engl J Med 2002; 347:956-62.

5. The impact of the erosion of retiree health benefits on workers and retirees. Issue brief. No. 279. Washington, D.C.: Employee Benefits Research Institute, March 2005. Available at: http://www.ebri.org/publications/ib/index.cfm?fa=ibDisp&content_id=3497 Accessed on August 6, 2007

6. Available at:

http://www.latimes.com/news/nationworld/nation/la-na-

gop6aug06,1,5334046.story?coll=la-headlines-nation&ctrack=1&cset=true Accessed on August 6, 2007

7. Available at:

http://online.wsj.com/article/SB118532549004277031.html?mod=djemHL Accessed on August 6, 2007

8. Available at:

http://www.oecd.org/document/10/0,3343,en_2649_201185_38976778_1_1_1_1,

00.html Accessed on August 6, 2007

9. Available at:

http://www.oecd.org/LongAbstract/0,3425,en_2649_201185_1862393_1_1_1_1,0

0.html Accessed on August 6, 2007

10. Available at:

http://www.ama-assn.org/amednews/2007/08/13/prl10813.htm Accessed on August 6, 2007

11. Kaul M. (1997). The New Public Administration: management innovation in government. Public Administration and Development. 17: 13-26.

12. Available at: http://www.cato.org/testimony/ct-dg06132007.html Accessed on August 10, 2007

13. Anderson GF. From 'Soak The Rich' To 'Soak The Poor': Recent Trends In Hospital Pricing Health Affairs, May/June 2007; 26(3): 780-789.

14. Available at:

http://seattletimes.nwsource.com/html/health/2002136353_fastfood31.html August 11, 2007.

15. Available at: http://www.kff.org/insurance/upload/7670.pdf Accessed on

August 11, 2007

16. Available at:

http://www.commonwealthfund.org/usr_doc/Collins_riteofpassage2007_1049

_ib.pdf?section=4039 Accessed on August 11, 2007

17. DeNavas-Walt C, Proctor BD, Lee CH, Income, Poverty, and Health Insurance Coverage in the United States: 2005, Current Population Reports, Consumer Income (Washington, D.C.: U.S. Census Bureau, Aug. 2006).

18. Mokdad AH, Ford ES, Bowman BA et al., "Prevalence of Obesity, Diabetes, and Obesity-Related Health Risk Factors, 2001," Journal of the American Medical Association, Jan. 1, 2003 289(1):76–79;

19. D. M. Mills, "The State of Student Health Insurance: Implications for ACHA's Standards," 2007 Student Health Insurance/Benefit Plan Survey Results, presentation at ACHA's Annual Meeting, Jun 1 2007.

20. Available at: Health Insurance Coverage: Early Release of Estimates from the

National Health Interview Survey, 2006 PDF (16 pages, 352 KB) Accessed on

August 12, 2007

21. Available at: Ambulatory Medical Care Utilization Estimates for 2005 PDF

(352 KB) Accessed on August 12, 2007

The Medicine-Technology Dyad in Health Insurance

It is paradoxical that progress in Technology and Medicine has often been the culprits in the soaring healthcare costs blame-game, typical of many contemporary health systems. Yet, we depend on such progress to improve healthcare delivery, prevent diseases, and save lives, all of which it indisputably also does. The issue then is how we could make it do one, the latter, and not the other, the former. This is more so as no country could afford to spending increasing percentages of its gross domestic product (GDP), as is currently the case with many, on health services, yet, could any ignore the immense benefits to the health of its peoples of medical and technological progress. Furthermore, increasing healthcare spending by many countries do not necessarily translate to better healthcare and could in fact result in fewer people having access to health services, which is anathema to developments in some countries presently regarding health insurance coverage, including the USA. In June 2007, the US Centres for Disease Control and Prevention's (CDC) National Centre for Health Statistics (NCHS) released selected estimates of health insurance coverage for the civilian non-institutionalized U.S. population based on data from the 2006 National Health Interview Survey (NHIS), alongside similar estimates from the 1997–2005 NHIS1. The estimates in 2006 showed the percentage of uninsured persons of all age groups being 14.8% (43.6 million) a significant increase over 2005, 16.8% (43.3 million) for individuals under the age of 65 years, 19.8% (36.5 million) for those aged 18–64 years, and 9.3% (6.8 million) for children under 18 years. A new Commonwealth Fund report, 'Rite of Passage - Why Young Adults Become Uninsured and How New Policies Can Help'2, notes that 13.3 million young adults between 19 to 29 years were uninsured in 2005, up from 12.9 million in 2004. The report also notes that young adults are still the largest age group without health insurance, and that being just 17 percent of the under-65 population regardless, in the group, they constitute 30 percent of the uninsured. Furthermore, 41% of uninsured young adults, ages 19-29 belongs to families below the poverty level, and the incomes of 72 percent are below twice the poverty level. No doubt, these figures are instructive, more so regarding young adults, and the reasons for the increase in the number of uninsured in the US are legion. Nonetheless, one cannot gainsay that efforts at dismantling the barriers to needed healthcare are crucial and indeed, urgent, in any country, given the vicious cycle of escalating health spending and worsening disease burden that lack of access to health services ultimately spawn. In other words, it is important to arrest increasing health spending not just because of its potential to compromise services provision of other sorts yet essential to the smooth operations of society, but also because not doing so, simply further increases the costs of health services provision. Thus, the overall result of escalating health spending, transcends the health domain, and could spell, potentially, economic, and social chaos. Given that medicine and technology are potent health cost drivers, at least in some respects, should we therefore, jettison the option of how they could become costs 'busters'? Could we not structure health insurance such that these two important scientific endeavours operate in tandem to facilitate as opposed to hinder access to required healthcare? Could the medicine-technology dyad not in fact, juxtapose with health insurance to form a veritable triangular interplay that opens up healthcare access, by keeping costs down, without compromising, and indeed actually improving the quality of care delivery? In other words, could this interplay not facilitate the achievement of these dual healthcare delivery objectives (DHDO) that would sooner than later actually be imperative for any health system to pursue? There is no doubt about the dire need of attention to expanding healthcare coverage in the US for example, considering the figures given above. Indeed, many states, sixteen since 2003, have passed laws to expand such coverage for dependent young adults up to 24 or 25 years old under parents' insurance policies2. Collins and her colleagues in the Commonwealth Fund report also mentioned earlier suggested three policy measures that could further assist uninsured young adults in acquiring coverage and prevent others from losing the coverage that they have2. They are, extending eligibility for public insurance programs past age 18; extending dependents' eligibility for their parents' private coverage past age 18 or 19; and ensuring that colleges not only oblige full- and part-time students to have coverage, but also offer them coverage2. Additionally, considering that most uninsured young adults have low wages, and may not be able to afford health insurance that in any case, their absence from the health risk pool partly accounts for soaring health insurance premiums costs, extending eligibility for Medicaid and the State Children's Health Insurance Program (SCHIP) beyond age 18 is crucial. This makes the SCHIP reauthorization bill that the House of Representatives recently passed, which enables states to extend coverage up to age 25, whereas Medicaid and SCHIP coverage for children characteristically stops at age 19 currently, apt. Yet, the issues involved in achieving or not the DHDO are way beyond simply ensuring access to healthcare. Indeed, addressing the issues pertaining to health services provision comprehensively is what any country, needs to achieve these dual objectives, as opposed to any 'automatic' measures, or presumed 'panacea' whose benefits would probably not just be transient, but which could in fact be counterproductive ultimately. What for example would an individual benefit from access to flawed care, and would such substandard or poor quality care not increase morbidity and overall disease burden for that individual and for the health system, further escalating costs? Why would a country not continue to spend increasing amounts of its national wealth on health that does not comprehend or acknowledge the legitimacy of the above questions, and their likely, rational answers, and prepare in addition to expanding coverage to accept, and tackle the challenges for example that the likely resulting moral hazard and adverse selection would pose? In other words, why would healthcare consumers not accept the responsibilities that come with such coverage expansion, if indeed, aware of them, or put differently, why would the health system, as part of acknowledging these and other challenges, not reward healthcare consumers who 'contribute' to the prospects of achieving the DHDO, and vice versa? True, we have introduced conditions such as 'if, indeed, aware of them,' that is the responsibilities that come with the expansion in coverage that made access to care possible for them, but that simply makes it mandatory that they do. In other words, part of the responsibility of the rest of us is to make those not aware of the need to avoid unhealthy lifestyles, to engage in physical exercise, to lose or gain weight to optimal levels, and to undergo cancer screening for examples, so to do. This explains the importance of incorporating for example the appropriate healthcare information and communication technologies (healthcare ICT) that could facilitate the process of information dissemination, in healthcare strategies considerations. In this instance, these technologies, and advancements in their varieties, could in effect, actually help reduce rather than increase healthcare costs, simultaneously improving health and health services delivery. Indeed, in emphasizing disease prevention and health promotion in their healthcare strategies, businesses would be shifting usage from 'costly high-tech' investigations/procedures to 'cheaper, but still high-tech' approaches that reduce health spending and assure health and well-being. This also underscores the importance of attention to the interplay of the triangle of medicine, technology, and health insurance mentioned earlier by businesses and indeed, other health services purchasers, and healthcare stakeholders. Here again, we should emphasize the complexity of the issues pointing to the next step of encouraging the adoption of the information so provided as it would be insufficient merely to provide information to accomplish health promotion and disease prevention, and indeed, any other initiatives aimed at achieving the DHDO. In this regard, advances in behavioural medicine for example applied, would help in the relevant behavioural modifications prescribed in the information provided, again, stressing the interplay of medical and technological progress in achieving goals that health insurance at least in part aims to achieve. A critical point to emphasize also here is the voluntary nature of the application of the information, and indeed, its acquisition in the first place. Thus, an underlying principle in the success or otherwise of any health initiative hinges on the fundamentals of our very existence, our individual liberty, the appreciation of whose significance in full, therefore, is crucial to the interplay of factors in healthcare delivery. These issues also further highlight the importance of ensuring that initiatives, for example coverage expansion, serve their intended purposes. In other words, what would be purpose mandating individual health insurance, if the individual would not use aspects of the services for example those aimed at health and wellness, or even if on treatment, comply with components of the treatment regimes? Indeed, would the health system, or even businesses not be better able to achieve the DHDO, embracing and acting appropriately on these concepts, in fact, investing in, and promoting, rather than shunning medical and technological research and advances, for example that would enhance the prospects of individuals/workers acting on relevant health information, for example.

Acting on health information, or taking rational decisions on health matters, which is a major aspect of the value of the information in the first place, crucially also pivots on costs. In fact, businesses would be keen to ensure that spiralling healthcare costs become history, and that costs do not compromise their ability to provide health insurance, specifically, qualitative healthcare coverage, to their employees. Yet, developments in the health insurance industry point to costs as one of the central players in the corporate healthcare delivery dynamics. According to the 2006 Employer Health Benefits Survey released on September 26, 2006[3], by the Kaiser Family Foundation (KFF) and the Health Research and Educational Trust (HRET), premiums for employer-sponsored health coverage increased an average 7.7 percent in 2006, even if less than the 9.2 percent increase recorded in 2005 and the recent peak of 13.9 percent in 2003. Despite that, 2006 showed the slowest premium growth rate until then since 2000, premiums still increased over twice as fast as workers' earnings (3.8 percent) and overall inflation (3.5 percent) did 3. Thus, workers are still paying more. Indeed, premiums have risen 87 percent over the previous six years to 2006, in which year family health coverage cost an average $11,480 per year, with workers paying averagely, $2,973 on premiums, about $1,354 more than in 2000[3]. This is clearly a recipe for workers, some at least, opting for compensation options in lieu of the increasing healthcare cost sharing that many businesses now increasingly offer, roughly two in five small businesses not even offering health insurance and those that do want workers on average to make much more contributions to their premiums, for example, for family coverage[3]. In effect, many workers do not have or are opting out of access to healthcare, which just as clearly does not bode well for either the worker or the firm. This makes it necessary if not in fact, urgent finding more appropriate solutions to the challenges of contemporary health services delivery, which businesses face, underscoring the need to examine what the medicine-technology dyad has to offer, among other options. To underline this point about costs further, the KFF/ HRET survey found enrollment in consumer-driven health plans (CDHP) to be modest, with 2.7 million workers in high-deductible plans with a savings option, those qualifying for Health Savings Accounts (HSAs) inclusive, just 4 percent of covered workers enrolled in such plans, similar to 2005 rates. In fact, only 7 percent of employers offering health benefits offer (CDHP) and very few firms offering other forms of insurance, expressed an interest in adopting in 2007, high-deductible plans that qualify for an HSA (4 percent) or linked with a Health Reimbursement Arrangement (6 percent). Could the role that costs play in the corporate health services equation be clearer given these figures regarding tax- favored accounts that employees could use to fund medical bills? Could workers be showing little interests in CDHPs because consumers pay directly for a larger share of their healthcare, even considering the potential incentive thereof for more rational service utilization, hence lower healthcare spending overall? Is this a matter of workers not appreciating in full the benefits derivable from such plans, and are firms, interestingly, 12 percent of firms with 1,000 or more workers offer an HSA-qualified plan, not showing interest because the workers are not, or for the same lack of understanding in full, of the significance of the underlying fundamental principles? There is no doubt that firms are exploring a variety of options as parts of their healthcare strategies, for example pay-for-performance (P4P), but the key objectives essentially remain the same, the DHDO. The question then is if these firms are exploring the fundamental principles upon which these various options hinge and if they coincided with those crucial to the success of their resultant initiatives in achieving the DHDO. A firm that opts for P4P for example would need to determine which patient outcome indicators are appropriate in evaluating provider performance, in particular given the variety of tasks and providers that could be part of the management of a particular patient. According to a recent study on which such indicators primary care physicians considered important components of a practice performance tool, 19 health characteristics emerged as important or very important4. They fit into eight domains: physical functioning, psychological functioning, social functioning, pain, quality of life, physiologic symptoms, health behaviours, and clinical indicators. The authors observed that notably absent were measures of social support and health perceptions, and recommended that such data as theirs should influence the development of practice performance measures. Indeed, it is important for businesses to be cognizant of developments in medicine, both in the clinical and management domains that could help tease out issues relating to which of CDHP, P4P, health savings accounts (HSA), disease-management approaches, and tiered-payments model, among other increasingly common models that employers embrace, in for example the US, to adopt. Also in the US, the Geisinger Health System's new approach to elective coronary-artery bypass grafting (CABG) is a case in point5. Essentially, Geisinger, an integrated health care delivery system in northeastern Pennsylvania, pledges to complete 40 key processes for every patient that undergoes elective CABG, albeit attainment of several of the "benchmarks" would be prior to or after hospitalization. Furthermore, even if Geisinger could not guarantee good clinical outcomes, its fees are a standard flat rate covering care for related complications during the 90 days post-surgery. Thus, the program would not charge additionally, except pre-existent, for treatment of sternal wound infections or heart failure consequent upon a perioperative infarction, if the patient received the care at a Geisinger facility5. The Geisinger program gained national prominence after a May 17, 2007, front-page article in the New York Times discussed it5, many hospitals now potentially keen to adopt the program, with its promise to provide an alternative to customary FFS care,

Selected Key Processes in the Geisinger "Proven Care" Elective CABG Program.*

Preadmission documentation
- American College of Cardiology–American Heart Association indication for surgery
- Explanation of treatment options to patient
- Indication of whether patient is a current user of clopidogrel or warfarin
- Screening for stroke risk
- Screening for use of epiaortic echocardiography

Operative documentation
- Patient receives correct dose of beta-blocker
- Patient receives preoperative antibiotics (within 60 minutes of incision; with vancomycin within 120 minutes)
- Left internal thoracic artery is used for grafting of the left anterior descending artery

Postoperative documentation
- Antibiotics are administered (postoperatively, for 24 to 48 hours)
- Beta-blocker is administered (within 24 hours after surgery)
- Tobacco screening and counseling are provided

Discharge documentation
- Referral to cardiac rehabilitation is provided
- Discharge medications (aspirin, beta-blockers, statin) are prescribed

Postdischarge documentation
- Patient is taking medications correctly
- Patient has or has not resumed smoking
- Patient is enrolled in cardiac rehabilitation

* CABG denotes coronary-artery bypass grafting.

In future, firms would likelier consider providers that operate on such defined evidence-based, principles, which would no doubt facilitate the realization of the DHDO, even if they would need, as would likely be the case, expert opinion on making such determinations, and regarding the potential contributions of advances in medicine and technology to their healthcare strategies. For example, that included in the guidelines are clear indications for the procedure, some of which require review by a colleague, even contra-indicate surgery, ensures that patients do not undergo them at the patients' or surgeon's whim, for whatever underlying reason, obviating the need for potentially unnecessary health spending. It is empowering for the patient though that a key preadmission benchmark is the mandatory review of treatment options by the surgeon with the patient, to ensure that the patient not only needs but also desires the procedure. The post-discharge benchmarks stress the responsibility that the patient has to ensuring the success of the operation for examples regarding follow-up and rehabilitation management programs. The Geisinger program also leaves room for some flexibility, to meet individual patient's needs, the surgeon, however, required to give cogent reasons, for deviating from the protocol, for example, deciding not to necessarily to use 'epiaortic echocardiography to screen for atheromata prior to operating on the aorta5'. Does that the Geisinger program has its own insurance company, the Geisinger Health System pays its doctors, it has a 'culture' and an efficient healthcare information system (HIS), not underline the point of our discussion regarding the potential benefits of the interplay of the medicine/technology/ health insurance triangle? Indeed, we also see with the example that within the context of an enabling culture of cooperation and receptivity to change the medicine/technology dyadic in tandem with health insurance could facilitate the realization of the DHDO. The point here is that businesses in designing their healthcare strategies need to have a broad perspective of the variables involved and their interplay, and to incorporate this understanding into their particular healthcare delivery options, within their peculiar health and economic milieus. There is no doubt about the increasing role that expertise, from within and outside the firm, would play for the analyses of these interlocking variables and their consequences for the company's strategic decision making on health services provision for its workers. This is more so as the changes in medicine, both from the clinical and management perspectives and in technology as they relate to these and other aspects of healthcare delivery would be ongoing, subject to advances in both fields. Experts for example contend that Geisinger's case rate and critical pathways approach would likely be the direction of P4P in future5. This is in contrast with current P4P models involving, for example, quality-of-care measures for patients with diabetes that focus on populations of patients who care primary care physicians manage5. In other words, the tendency for P4Pwould be not just rewarding volume as incentives would need to be stronger and more focused, and would be applicable to not just surgical procedures, but also diseases such as high blood pressure, diabetes, asthma, cancer, and indeed, all others, and to the activities of every healthcare professional involved in the care provision. Thus, healthcare providers, health plans, and other insurers would increasingly link incentives to such individual patient management predicated on evidence-based critical pathways of care that would be subject to measurement and evaluation, and which would thus likely ensure improved outcomes. They would also, cognizant of medical progress, evaluate appropriately, changes in the practice of providers, with not just cost implications, but that could potentially save the lives of their workers. Consider for example, a recent study published in the August 15, 2007 issue of the Journal of the American Medical Association (JAMA) 6, which found that the lipid measure apolipoprotein (apo) B: apo A-I ratio is not a better predictor of coronary heart disease risk than traditional lipid ratios that include total cholesterol and HDL-C. Presently, risk-prediction instruments and guidelines for coronary heart disease (CHD) prevention stress the use of low-density lipoprotein cholesterol (LDL-C), total cholesterol, or both for CHD risk assessment. However, in recent years, evidence has shown up suggesting that higher apo B, the primary protein part of LDL, and lower apo A-I, the primary protein part of high-density lipoprotein [HDL, levels play a role in the development of CHD, and that these measures might be superior to customary lipid measures for CHD risk prediction. According to the authors of this study, "Our principal findings are 3-fold. First, even though the apo B:apo A-I ratio performed well overall in terms of CHD risk prediction and model performance measures in both sexes, the differences compared with other lipid variables were small and statistically nonsignificant. Non-HDL-C performed relatively less well compared with the lipid ratios. Second, when CHD risk reclassification was evaluated, the differences in net reclassification improvement offered by the total cholesterol: HDL-C ratio vs. the apo B: apo A-I ratio was small and statistically nonsignificant in both sexes. Third, the apo B:apo A-I ratio was not significantly associated with CHD incidence in either sex when added to a model that incorporated components of the Framingham risk score, including total cholesterol:HDL-C. This observation suggests that apo B: apo A-I ratio does not provide incremental predictive utility over established CHD risk factors including traditional lipid measures." In other words, apolipoproteins, the protein component of serum lipoproteins, are not superior to traditional lipid measures for CHD risk prediction, and indeed, may be costlier to use in some instances. As the authors also noted, "Given overall equal performance of various lipids ratios, other factors will be critical in guiding the choice of lipid measures that should be used for CHD risk prediction. These factors include the costs and availability of assays, educational needs for health care professionals, and the public for interpreting apolipoprotein measures, the possibility of obtaining valid measurements for risk prediction in nonfasting samples, or in patients receiving lipid-lowering treatment, and the availability of appropriate therapeutic cut-points and clinical evidence of benefits accruing from lowering levels (based on randomized, controlled clinical trials). However, with regard to test performance characteristics, our data do not support the need for measuring apo B or apo A-I in clinical practice when traditional lipid measurements are obtained routinely." Of potential interest to firms, providers, and insurers, would also likely be another study published in the same edition of the journal that also looked at the apolipoproteins, this time at the increasing interests in high-density lipoprotein cholesterol (HDL-C), a cardiovascular risk factor, as a therapeutic target7. The authors reviewed the current and emerging strategies that modify high-density lipoproteins (HDLs), and concluded that 'at present there is modest evidence to support aggressively increasing HDL-C levels in addition to what is achieved by lifestyle modification alone.Ongoing clinical trials that target specific pathways in HDL metabolism may help expand cardiovascular treatment options.' These two related examples show the significance for practice, and for treatment outcomes, and costs, attention to medical progress could be, something that firms would appreciate ever more in the days ahead. As part of ensuring that, the implications of these research findings trickle down on critical decision making regarding health services utilization, hence improve services delivery quality, and reduce costs, firms would need to design initiatives appropriate to their organizations for their workers too. For example, they would need to ensure that their workers also receive the relevant research information, in ways understandable to them, which by the way, they appropriate use of the right information and communication technologies, could help with, and perhaps more importantly, act on it. With regards these technologies, incidentally, the increasing appreciation of their potential to 'revolutionize' medical practice and health insurance is evident in the entrepreneurial vigour increasingly infused into healthcare. Indeed, these technologies would not only help focus more on achieving the dual healthcare delivery objectives, but also on reducing costs and improving care quality, and indeed, on empowering patients. Perot Systems for example in Mid-August 2007 announced it purchased JJWild of Canton, Massachusetts for US$89 million. JJWild is the preferred system integrator for the MEDITECH system, used in 2,000 hospitals, the system developed and marketed by Medical Information Technology, Inc. With financial backing from Steve case, AOL founder, Revolution Health, which plans to incorporate social networking and personalization into WebMD and Healthline, for examples, is another example, and there are many more. Firms, in ensuring the realization of the DHDO would be showing increasing interests in the applications of technological innovations in medicine and in understanding the surplus of choices even healthcare providers that have embraced these technologies face. In other words, just as the providers and other healthcare stakeholders would, firms would need to fathom what the innovations do, which ones particular providers need to adopt, routinely, and optionally, for examples, and which ones would benefit their workers, for example, regarding health education and promotion, or disease monitoring, at work. As with keeping up with the advances in medicine and taking such crucial decisions regarding their choices of providers, or what to expect of them, and regarding the company's healthcare strategy at large, firms might need expert opinion, from within the firm, or via an external consultant. These experts would need to conduct analyses of these issues on an ongoing basis in order that the firms would have updated information on which to base what should be ongoing reviews of their healthcare strategies as well. Firms, in consultation with expert opinion would need to work with care providers on the relevant issues in ICT deployment, examining the potential contributions of these technologies to improving service delivery considering their classification into three broad categories for example. These categories are function ICT, which includes technologies, for example, word processors, and spreadsheets applications that improve the efficiency of individual tasks; and network ICT that includes those applications that facilitate communication, for examples e-mail, instant messaging (IM), and even electronic newsletters, web information portals, and blogs. A third group comprises enterprise IT, with a focus on customer resource management and supply chain management that improves interactions within the firm, and between it and its associates, such as clients and suppliers. Firms in fact would need to adopt such an approach to evaluating the technologies that their providers not only currently use, but also propose to implement in their quest to continue to improve efficiency in health services delivery, which among others, would translate overall into the firm achieving the DHDO regarding its healthcare strategy.

The transformations that are ongoing in medicine we contend have important ramifications for the future of both healthcare delivery and of access to it. Given the two fundamental economic principles that society cannot meet all the needs of everyone all the time, and that resources are scarce anyway, the need for resource optimization would continue to be crucial in any healthcare delivery efforts, either from the perspective of public or private health financing. Thus, the need to marry developments in medicine and technology in making health insurance more affordable, the quality of health services better, and the costs of providing these services lesser, is indeed, imperative, regardless of the financing model in question. Indeed, health systems would increasingly realize the benefits to their survival of embracing this seemingly complex, comprehensive, although actually relatively simpler, vis-à-vis the 'confusion' that mars current efforts at health sector reform (HSR) in many countries, model. In other words, health services delivery would no longer simply be a matter of expanding coverage as such expansion, in itself does not guarantee qualitative services, which guarantee is crucial to the expansion, realistically, as increased morbidity could only lead to reduced capacity for expansion eventually, hence, and more importantly would be expansion in tandem with quality and cost-effectiveness. It is clear then that neither the private nor public sector could ignore for too long, the importance of being cognizant of medical and technological advances for the success or otherwise of healthcare delivery efforts. This is not to diminish the significance of access to health, which as a recent study that aimed to examine whether patients with no insurance or Medicaid are more likely to present with advanced-stage laryngeal cancer, showed, is significant in many respects[8]. The authors conducted a retrospective cohort study from the US National Cancer Database, 1996-2003. They found patients with advanced-stage laryngeal cancer at diagnosis likelier to be uninsured or covered by Medicaid compared with those with private insurance. They also found that patients were likeliest to present with the largest tumours (T4 disease) if they were uninsured or covered by Medicaid, and that patients who were black, between 18 and 56 years old, and lived in zip codes with low percentages of high school graduates or low median household incomes likelier received advanced disease and/or larger tumours-diagnosis. The authors concluded that persons that lack insurance or on Medicaid are at most risk for presenting with advanced laryngeal cancer, and suggested the probable effect of post-diagnosis enrolment of the uninsured on the Medicaid group results. They also noted the importance of considering the effect of insurance coverage on stage at diagnosis and associated morbidity, mortality, quality of life, and costs. Indeed, addressing the complexity of the elements of health and healthcare delivery, both health and non-health related, successfully, requires the simplicity, paradoxically, inherent in applying the decomposition/exposition exercises contingent upon the ongoing process cycle analyses of the medicine-technology dyad. In fact, firms even now, should no longer ignore for example, the potential effects on their healthcare goals of research findings such as those mentioned above in relation to laryngeal cancer. This is more so as these findings might apply to other diseases, and underscore the need for just as eclectic the conceptualization of the underlying factors in disease causation, and outcome as the approaches to tackling them. As the authors noted, for example, individuals with laryngeal cancer might just be entering the health system a little late was why many more had late-stage and larger cancers under Medicaid, as the situation with those uninsured seems clear enough. Yet, it is apt to ask the question why they entered Medicaid late to begin with or perhaps if the services Medicaid offers are inferior to those received by persons with private insurance. It is perhaps plausible to surmise that both factors were operational, and perhaps even more, such as why some individuals were uninsured in the first place. The point here is that we should learn some lessons regarding the insights we could imbibe from medical research to support our approaches to health services delivery that might otherwise be lacking due to political and other exigencies. It would be difficult to justify the actions taken counter to the ramifications deducible from these researches, some of which could be far-reaching in terms of the survival, let alone progress of our establishments, and by extension, even ourselves, even if in the long term. Thus, a firm would see the desirability in ensuring that its workers do not opt for juicer, that is financially, alternative compensation packages in lieu of contributing higher proportions of their healthcare bills, for example. Nor would it encourage even tacitly, the exclusion from the health risk pool of some of its higher-paid, and healthier employees, leaving adjusting premiums higher until they could do so no more, and run out of business, even if only because the cascading effects of soaring healthcare costs that ensue due to increased morbidity. This is likely going to be so due to the large numbers of the already attenuated individuals left in the pool. Meanwhile, some of those hitherto healthy would also become ill at some point but might be avoiding required care because they have shunned health insurance, hence enter health services late, and at more expense, the disease burden that results from both groups clearly unlikely to be favourable to their employers overall. Similar issues would arise as genetic medicine for example, becomes more prominent in medical practice as the intricacies of extrapolating for instance clinical practice from organic molecules become increasingly resolved. Here is another example of the interface between medicine and technology yielding crucial insights into determinations in health insurance, for example pricing, equally germane to not just the progress, if not in fact the survival of both the health and insurance industries, but also of businesses. As scientists continue to explore biological and medica informatics, it would be possible for example to have an individual's health and disease profiles. Indeed, genetic profiles might be available for an individual right from birth detailing his or her predisposition to certain diseases, and health problems, which might help determine health risks and ways to mitigate them. Employers, for example, would increasingly evaluate in future, their employees' physical and psychological health and risk factors for illnesses, more so evident in their genetic profiles. They would likely request such profiles as the technologies become available and accessible for doing so, perhaps not so much to exclude some individuals from employment, but to take the necessary measures to preempt age-related diseases, for example, reduce the damage to health of others, as part of the strategic healthcare initiatives to keep their workers healthy. In other words, firms would increasingly embrace a variety of models of healthcare appropriate to their particular settings, including, which most should, and probably would, the population health model of primary, secondary, and tertiary prevention. Thus, firms would be current on the approaches to preventing diseases from starting to begin with, and once they do, to ensure their prompt diagnosis and effective treatment, and indeed, to ensure the proper management of their complications, including rehabilitation in different respects, physical, mental, and vocational, for examples, among others. These three pillars of disease prevention would, also increasingly involve the combined insights from medical and technological progress, whose effects on the nature and type of health services used would no doubt profoundly affect the health insurance industry, not just in terms of the services and products they and healthcare providers offer, but also their pricing. These developments would hence also affect the healthcare consumer, in terms of affordability of health insurance, and accessibility to care among others, which in relation to firms, would affect their abilities to realize the DHDO, for example, and the productivity of their workers, hence the businesses' bottom line. There is no doubt about the future of healthcare likely being predicated on principles such as we have here discusses, in particular on the need for process cycle analyses, which would expose the issues and their parts involved in healthcare delivery in a particular jurisdiction, hence the potential solutions to them. In using the term jurisdiction broadly, we acknowledge the pervasive nature of healthcare issues and the applicability of many of the principles important to addressing these issues successfully in different domains. Thus, it is important for all healthcare stakeholders to strive to achieve the dual healthcare delivery objectives (DHDO), for example, yet the approaches to so doing would be different given the peculiarities of each stakeholder's respective jurisdiction. In the same vein, every healthcare stakeholder would need to be conversant with developments in medicine and technology, with a view to incorporating those relevant to their needs in their respective approaches to health services delivery or utilization. It is also an important generic principle that we could never expect these activities to be perfect, as the share variety of elements involved in the healthcare delivery enterprise makes it Herculean, literally, to expect all to operate perfectly and in unison all the time. Indeed, we this possible, the health system is inherently imperfect, due to the imperative of change, as occasioned for examples, by medical and technological progress. It is thus in fact, imperative that firms, and indeed, all healthcare stakeholders embrace these generic and specific principles, as change would impel their applicability, anyway, and those of others, which would emerge given the particular state of affairs in question. Put differently, it would be foolhardy for a firm not to pay attention to changes in medicine and technology, which incidentally, could operate singly or together to result in sometimes-paradigmatic shifts in medical practice of seismic proportions, literally, with potent ramifications for healthcare costs, and the nature and quality of service delivery. Indeed, it would be ever more the hallmark of the successful firm that is able not just to be aware, fully appreciate the implications of, and incorporate in its healthcare strategy on an ongoing basis, progress in medicine and technology, to create, in fact, novel initiatives that would differentiate it, and enhance its competitiveness, rather than drain its bank accounts. In other words, strategic corporate healthcare philosophy would become not a nuisance but an asset, in some cases, a core competence, which others would indeed, attempt to emulate. At this level, it would not just enable the firm realize its goals of a healthy workforce with costs kept at reasonable minimum, but the initiatives emergent from the strategies for example would empower its workers, engender a sense of belonging and ownership of the firm, foster employee loyalty, and improve productivity. These attributes would be evident in not just its turnover as a direct consequence of its increased productivity, but also in its increasing patronage that the improved customer relations that a healthy and happy workforce generates. Thus, as is the case at the individual level, the conceptualization of healthcare delivery would become more comprehensive, and firms, and indeed, other healthcare stakeholders would actively pursue well-thought-out healthcare strategies that serve their interests and those of their employees, rather than just theirs. This trend would be actually the inevitable outcome of changes both within and without the health system, many already under way, which would be and those already ongoing are clearly the antithesis of societal progress, something few would argue is not critical to our continued survival as a species. It is obvious for example that foot and mouth disease on a farm in a remote English town, could result in the immediate slaughtering of millions of cows in neighbouring towns and indeed, in the entire country, and worse still, the banning of importation of cows from the country by others worldwide. The devastation to the livelihoods of the farmers and to the country's economy could be immense. Indeed, these losses could boomerang on the availability of funds for the country's National Health Service (NHS), compromise its people's health, and further, by reducing productivity, its economy. This is not to mention that the disease could be one that not only affects the animals but like Mad cow's disease, humans who ate meat from infected cows. Firms would also be showing interests in their workers' health and being profitable and surviving being involved in their respective jurisdictions in ways supportive of progress in healthcare delivery, and not otherwise. Hence, it would unlikely be the case as recently suspected to be so in the UK with the outbreak of foot-and mouth-disease in Surrey that a private firm, incidentally working on a vaccine to prevent the disease was the likely source of its outbreak. The link of the damage to human health resultant were this in fact the case between the activities of the firm that led to the outbreak, and this damage might indeed, seem tenuous, but these flaws add up, as is evident in the outcome of many years of folly in healthcare administration in many countries today. These outcomes by the way have had major effects on some of the major firms in the world, for example, General Motors, bothering on financial ruin. To be sure, some would blame the firms for their lack of foresight in offering those generous post WWII compensation packages, even though that shoddiness with which successive governments handles the emergent power of the health insurance industry, coupled with the supply-side spending spree in which they engaged, among other follies, should not also take the blame is moot. It is ironical though that the 'markets giants' in Detroit did not envisage the awesome power of the market in shaping developments even in the health sector, and the role that they needed to play in not just job creation, but in deploying the necessary measures as the 'saga' of health services delivery unfolds over the years. This is why all firms and not just the big ones should not miss the chance to engage actively in this change process. Part of so doing involves, as we have observed here, taking the matter of their strategic healthcare strategy seriously. The point is that firms cannot afford gerrymandering with this matter, given that their very survival is at stake, as is that of the economy, and of course ultimately, the polity. Given that their constituency is in a sense limited, their shareholders, yet diverse in another, their clients, businesses have the advantage over politicians of harnessing this eclectic leverage in spearheading appropriate initiatives in their jurisdictions to foster healthcare delivery, primarily among their workers, but also the populace at large. Firms would need and urgently too, to reorient their worldview of health services along the lines we have discussed among others, acknowledging such services as purveyors of pervasive developments within their firms, and in society in general.

References:

1. Cohen RA, Martinez ME. Health insurance coverage: Early release of estimates from the National Health Interview Survey, 2006. June 2007.
Available at: http://www.cdc.gov/nchs/nhis.htm. Accessed on August 12, 2007

2. Collins SR, Schoen C, Kriss JL, Doty MM, Mahato B. Rite of Passage? Why Young Adults Become Uninsured and How New Policies Can Help, The Commonwealth Fund, Updated August 8, 2007

3. Available at: http://www.kff.org/insurance/ehbs092606nr.cfm Accessed on August 13, 2007

4. Dassow, Paul L. Measuring Performance in Primary Care: What Patient Outcome Indicators Do Physicians Value? Journal of the American Board of Family Medicine. 20(1):1-8, January/February 2007.

5. Lee TH. Pay for Performance, Version 2.0? New England Journal of Medicine. 357(6):531-533, August 9, 2007.

6. Ingelsson E, Schaefer EJ, Contois JH, McNamara, JR, Sullivan L, Keyes MJ,

et.al. Clinical Utility of Different Lipid Measures for Prediction of Coronary Heart Disease in Men and Women. JAMA. 298(7):776-785, August 15, 2007.

7. Singh IM, Shishehbor MH, Ansell BJ. High-Density Lipoprotein as a Therapeutic Target: A Systematic Review. JAMA. 298(7):786-798, August 15, 2007

8. Chen AY, Schrag NM, Halpern M, Stewart A, Ward EM. Health Insurance and Stage at Diagnosis of Laryngeal Cancer: Does Insurance Type Predict Stage at Diagnosis? Arch Otolaryngol Head Neck Surg. 2007; 133:784-790.

The Future of Employer-Sponsored Health Insurance

Many would argue for scrapping employer-sponsored health insurance, that it does not work, evident in the US for example, by the large numbers of uninsured workers. Others would insist that it is the best option not just for providing healthcare to workers, but in the overall effort to improve the health system in many countries, if not even to keep it going to begin with. Given the passion cloaking these and other intermediate positions on employer-sponsored health insurance, it is apt to ask what its future is, in itself, and indeed, as an element of the private health insurance industry. It is also pertinent to ask how this industry would emerge from its present imbroglio with public health insurance as alternative health financing schemes, over which is superior and indeed, desirable, to affirm that passion is brewing is indeed, benign, considering the intensity of the divisions in the polity, over the issues involved. The Los Angeles Times recently reported that 'Gov. Arnold Schwarzenegger took a firm stand Wednesday against the Democratic healthcare proposal moving through the Legislature, saying for the first time that he would not support an expansion of medical insurance if it were financed solely by new requirements on employers1'. The paper added,' The Democratic proposal would require employers to spend at least the equivalent of 7.5% of their payroll on their workers' health. The governor insisted that the plan also must require all Californians to have insurance, an idea at the core of his January proposal.' Large corporations such as Wal-Mart are in league with the Service Employees International Union, a major Labor organization, in favor of universal coverage. In April 2007, an alliance of unions, firms, and foundations launched the 'Cover the Uninsured Week' campaign, with the aim of providing health insurance to all uninsured Americans. Heated political debates in the U.S Congress and Senate are underway, as they are on the campaign trails of presidential aspirants. The scale and complexity of these issues are, indeed, enormous. Yet, are we anywhere near their resolution? Besides such issues as the returns on expansion for equitability, which many would contend it would reduce, if not eliminate, although that it would, intra-demographic, say between young and elderly males, is less certain, questions regarding that for quality remain vexing. The real question though is not the issues that remain unresolved with coverage expansion, but whether those issues need persist at all, and if not, if universal coverage would eliminate them, or if indeed, employer-sponsored health insurance would be at the core of any measure that ultimately would. Could we in fact, be coupling healthcare financing too hard to service provision to the exclusion to a more or less extent of the more fundamental issues on which the success of the latter hinges? Hacker, in an article in the August 23, 2007 issue of the New England Journal of Medicine2 noted a recent Consumer Reports survey3 that shows about 50% of adults less than 65 years old, the majority insured, saying they are 'somewhat' or 'completely' not ready to cope with an expensive medical emergency in the year ahead. He also notes that a significant percentage, up to 50%, of the over 1 million personal bankruptcies in the US yearly, each year result partly from medical costs and crises, 4 and that nowhere else in the developed world are individuals anywhere as prone to report difficulty paying medical bills or shunning care for lack of funds5. Hacker not only also notes that the problems 'are long-standing-yes, "dating back to the 1980s"-and worsening,' but also that 'they are largely due to our reliance on employment-based, voluntary private health insurance'2.

Elsewhere in the article, Hacker notes, 'this is the catch-22 of health care reform: it is the very failings of our insurance system that make dealing with those failings so devilishly hard,' and essentially extolled Medicare, as 'the country's most popular and successful public insurance plan.' He added, 'Yet it has controlled expenses better than the private sector, spends little on administration, and allows patients to seek care from nearly every doctor and hospital.' It is doubtful that Medicare has all these flowery attributes6, and Hacker's suggestion that businesses either provide their employees 'with good private coverage or enrol them, at a modest cost, in a new public program modelled after Medicare,' echoes the dichotomization in health financing that we here emphasize is, and would become increasingly obvious over time, indeed is, redundant. Regarding businesses' current tendency to avoid health insurance, Hacker notes that this 'strategy would ensure that their retreat results not in greater dislocation and insecurity but in increasing numbers of Americans, gaining access to a national, Medicare-like plan that guarantees affordable, high quality care'7. Indeed, Hacker's suggestion that such a plan is akin to 'the one public program that most resembles the "free universal health care",' underscores his position that 'the Medicare model is the not-so-secret weapon in the campaign for affordable health care for all,' but is Medicare really the panacea? Documentation on Medicare's problems is legion. According to a 2005 USATODAY article6, "Social Security's fiscal problems would escalate in about 2018, when it is projected to begin paying out more in benefits than it receives in taxes; Medicare reached that milestone last year (2004)." At that time, over 41 million Americans depended on Medicare to pay for their doctors' visits and hospital bills, and in 2006, it also paid part of their prescription-drug bills, a program projected to cost over $700 billion over a decade. With Medicare, projected to grow by 9% a year through 2015, and Social Security's annual growth rate, an estimated 5.6%, the difference vis-à-vis the estimated general inflation growth rate of 3.2% is instructive6, the model applied to workers, and indeed, all Americans. Questions naturally arise where the funds would come from, with the country's population aging, among other issues, not to mention those relating to the quality of care delivered, which latter, if poor, could only open a revolving door of increasing morbidity and soaring healthcare costs, hence spending. Furthermore, it is uncertain how even if as Hacker noted, 'No doubt many employers would seize the opportunity to obtain inexpensive coverage for their workers, which would give the new public insurance plan a large, diverse enrolment,' this would offer 'a great deal of leverage to contain costs and improve care,' given the underlying moral hazard issues that would likely ensue. So is it not definite how, 'employers could also implement their own cost-control and quality-enhancement strategies, without having to bear the burden of uncompensated charity care for the uninsured and underinsured.' Indeed, these are issues, which would likely soar healthcare spending rather than the other way round, and to worsen matters, ultimately compromise the quality of care. With past efforts to enable Medicare considering costs in determining 'reasonable and necessary' care, which it covers by law, not successful, reducing waste and overuse of resources with this model is clearly likely going to keep being a chore. With the latest data released by the U.S. Census Bureau on August 28, 2007, showing that the number of uninsured Americans has increased to 47 million in 2006, from 44.8 million in 2005, as has the number of uninsured children, that the need to address the coverage issue in the country, is evident8. Indeed, the data revealed that both the percentage and the number of people without health insurance increased in 2006, the percentage without health insurance increased from 15.3 percent in 2005 to 15.8 percent in 2006. The data also showed that the number of individuals with health insurance rose to 249.8 million in 2006 (up from 249.0 million in 2005), and that the number of persons covered by private health insurance (201.7 million) and the number of those covered by government health insurance (80.3 million) were not statistically different in 2006 from 2005. Significantly, however, the percentage of people covered by employment-based health insurance decreased to 59.7 percent in 2006, from

60.2 percent in 2005, which raises the question regarding whether this reflects a pattern, and that would persist long into the future or if it would be temporary, and underlines the point about the need to address the issues involved in such decline. In fact, that the percentage of people covered by government health programs decreased to 27.0 percent in 2006 from 27.3 percent in 2005, highlights the urgency of the matter, even if the percentage and the number of people covered by Medicaid were statistically unchanged at 12.9 percent and 38.3 million, respectively, in 2006. This is more so, among other reasons, given the ramifications for overall healthcare costs not to mention disease burden being likely adverse in the long term, not just for the individual, businesses, but also the entire economy. Still in the U.S., it is also instructive that, as a recent nationwide survey of 1,557 employers conducted by Mercer Health & Benefits, showed 9, healthcare benefit costs for U.S. employers may increase an average of 6.7% to $8,500 per employee in 2008, versus the 6.1 percent another Mercer survey predicted for 2007, although nowhere near the double-digit increases the decade heralded, topped by a 14.7 percent increase in 200210. Indeed, the Mercer projection is that health plan costs would rise 9 percent for 2008, 9 with firms making no changes to their insurance plans, which explains why preliminary results of the survey shows over 50% of the respondents are looking at cost shifting to employees for examples via higher co-payments, deductibles, out-of-pocket maximums, or premiums. More specifically, the preliminary results indicate that 36% of employers intend to increase the percentage of premiums employees pay, 29% expect to increase deductibles, co-payments or the maximum out-of-pocket payments allowed employees, firms, changes that would result in a projected premiums' increase in 2008 of just 6.7 percent.. he question of health costs increasing or of whether employer-sponsored health coverage would account more for healthcare coverage in the U.S., and indeed, in other countries, including those now deemed to have predominantly publicly-financed health systems is indeed moot. The observation of Blaine Bos, a senior Mercer consultant in Minneapolis, "Employer thinking on what constitutes a 'fair share' for employees has definitely changed over the past few years," adding "But in many cases, we're seeing employers providing more choice rather than just shifting cost, so that employees have the opportunity to save money by selecting lower levels of coverage, 9" underlines this apparent paradox. His point also is in fact, significant to the final common pathway that would see employer-sponsored health insurance wax rather than wane. Indeed, the earlier Mercer survey referred to above also found that more employers are utilizing consumer-driven health plans, low-premium, high-deductible plans with health savings accounts, and disease prevention programs as cost-management strategies10. In other words, firms do not and really should not consider their workers' health trivial, perhaps as much as they do not want to run out of business. The question then is finding a meeting point where firms would be able to preserve and indeed, promote their workers' health, simultaneously, saving costs, for both, what we would regard as seeking the dual healthcare delivery objectives (DHDO.) According to this survey, 6% of employers offered consumer-driven plans in 2006, three times the percentage in 2005, and another 14% of employers are planning to offer consumer-driven plans in 2007, most preferring health savings accounts (HSAs) to health reimbursements accounts, which latter calls for contribution by employers11. Significantly, that the survey found that six in 10 small employers offered a consumer-driven plan as their only insurance option, compared with one in 10 large employers, that about 25% of employers offered preventive screenings in 2006, and that the percentage of large employers offering preventive screenings has almost doubled in the past three years, are instructive11. There is no doubt therefore of the potential for finding the common ground between employers and their workers that would at least keep employer-sponsored health insurance going. It is in fact likely to become increasingly clear that it has immense potential to address successfully many of the problems that plague many a health system in the world today. In other words, rather than become moribund, many health jurisdictions would in fact increasingly embrace employer-sponsored health insurance. The reasons for this development would hinge on those generic, and on others, more specific to particular health jurisdictions yet relatable to those generic. It might seem counterintuitive that employer-based health insurance would survive, let alone thrive in the U.S for example, given the seemingly ever-increasing premiums, which many firms, particularly the smaller firms and their workers find increasingly difficult to cope with, particularly as noted in a report released on September 11, 2007 by the Kaiser Family Foundation "Survey of Employer Benefits 2007" showing that since 2001, the cost of premiums has increased 78 percent, far outpacing a 19 percent wage increase and 17 percent inflation hike, with between 1 million and 2 million people becoming uninsured yearly12. In 2007, premiums averaged $12,106 for a family of four, out of which workers paid an average, $3,281, premiums for a single individual, $4,479, of which employers paid, $694. However, as also noted above, it is instructive that the increased premiums this year represent the lowest growth rates since 1999's 5.3%, the slowing in growth rates in the fourth consecutive year this year even if they are still 'growth" and workers are paying more as the growth outpaces wages and inflation, particularly with more firms shunning health insurance for their workers as a result12. The point remains though that we need therefore to examine in totality the root causes of the increasing premiums to stem their ramifications, including the increasing numbers of uninsured Americans, according to the Census Bureau estimates 15.8% in 2006, up from 15.3% in 20058. The question of whether insurance firms have been increasing premiums to expand or preserve profit margins for example is pertinent. In other words, are insurance companies charging more to cover what they pay out in claims, and if so, why are claims increasing? Should we not be examining the roles the lengthening duration of hospital stays, and hence costs, or the propensity for cutting-edge, but costly treatment options, or of expensive and hi-tech investigations, among others are playing in driving costs and claims? Should we in fact not be considering the reasons for these putative cost drivers and reducing their impact, which underscores the need for, among others, process cycle analysis, a decomposition/exposition exercise that would reveal the approaches to the relevant issues that could facilitate the achievement of the DHDO? What are the prospects of the private sector for example being better able to improve the efficiency and effectiveness of health services delivery based on the outcomes of such exercises compared to the public sector? These questions raise the spectre of the neglect that health systems around the world have suffered being perpetuated or not, depending on the realization or otherwise of the need to embrace the approaches to reorienting their motion via strict adherence to the principles of efficiency and cost-effectiveness. This in fact is not to condemn the public sector to oblivion in this regard, but an acknowledgement of the neglect, and a call to the operations of the public sector to improve their operations. More importantly though, are issues regarding the nature and extent of the involvement of the public sector in healthcare delivery in the first place. In other words, should this role properly be as a constituent of free-market operations, an essential option for the healthcare consumer, from which employers could purchase health services for their workers? The Kaiser survey mentioned above noted that 158 million persons receive employer-sponsored healthcare coverage, which 60% of firms provide in 2007, versus 69% in 2000, almost all firms with 50 or more employees offering coverage, but just 45% with three to nine employees do, versus 57% in 200012. If many firms are indeed, not contemplating dropping health insurance for their workers in 2008, but rather examining ways to make it affordable, the point we stress here about the likelihood of employer-sponsored health insurance actually waxing becomes more probable. In other words, these firms are unlikely to continue to offer health insurance to their workers if it would sink the firms literally, hence they would likelier seek ways to make it work for both themselves and for their workers, and indeed retirees. Is it any wonder then that democratic presidential candidate Hillary Rodham Clinton on Monday, September 17, 2007 noted, regarding her proposed health care reform plan to ensure coverage for all Americans, "I know my Republican opponents will try to equate health care for all Americans with government-run health care. Don't let them fool us again. This is not government-run." Alternatively, is it that her aides observed that she now favours a plan that emphasizes "simplicity, cost control and consumer choice?" 13 Criticisms of her idea of an 'individual mandate' regardless, her plan'American Health Choices Plan' aims to build on the current employer-based healthcare coverage system, with individuals on such insurance able to continue so to do, firms required to offer it, or contribute to a government-run pool to fund services for those not covered, a tax subsidy offered small businesses to ease costs burden. The plan also aims to offer scaled-up versions of two current government programs, namely Medicare, and the health insurance plan at present provided federal employees, as options from which the consumers could choose either, to persons and families employers do not cover, or cover inadequately. Besides the issues of the ethics of ending tax cuts to persons earning over $250,000 per year, one way anticipated for funding the plan, while giving others subsidy, the plan, no doubt raises those of the nature and extent of government involvement in healthcare delivery, which its core principle, that of an 'individual mandate' also emphasized, in particular in relation to the right of the individual to choose. This is not to mention, regarding the latter concern, how compliance with such a mandate would be different from that of the picture with auto insurance for example, which many drivers do not have, including the difficulty enforcing it. Yet, would we turn such persons back from the emergency room (ER) for example, if they showed up their after a collision, lacking not just auto insurance but also health insurance? These issues underscore the underpinnings of the preference for the adoption of a non-coercive approach to health insurance coverage, the success of which would require an appreciation of the fundamentals of such an approach that would result in the realization of the potential of employer-based health insurance being the pivotal option in health services provision, not just one that would make little or no difference to the exposition of the options and their hierarchy.

Thus, there would be complementary options, but it would be necessary to appreciate their relative significance and the dynamics between them. It is instructive for example to know the implications of the fundamental approach to health services delivery that does not exclude the contributions of public financing of health systems, despite that it acknowledges that employer-sponsored health coverage is the direction the health system should, and would indeed, move in the future. This is because for one, the public sector employs people, as does the private sector. In other words, those employers in the public sector would also need to provide health services to their workers, funded with public money. In other words, we cannot totally exclude the use of tax-payers funds to provide health services to people as matters currently stand in many, if not all countries. The question is whether we should and would need to reduce the size of the public sector to reduce this involvement or whether and as would likelier happen along with this downsizing, the public sector should 'behave' more like the private sector. In other words, should government employees be free to choose between attending a government-run hospital, assuming that government is still running hospitals, or a private hospital? If government was still running hospitals, should these hospitals not run as a private enterprise does, and if they did, what effect would this have on our understanding of, and approach to health services delivery? The point we are making here is that even government-run hospitals would have to operate as though they are in the free market, and the gearing of policy toward this situation would only facilitate inevitability. Thus, government-run hospitals would also to need to become more efficient and cost-effective to survive let alone thrive, and by giving their workers the option to attend government-run or private hospitals, the public sector would be facilitating the efficient running of these hospitals, which would not only save costs, and reduce health spending, but would also improve the quality of service provision. The alternative would be for them to become moribund in the face of stiff competition by hospitals in the private sector. In other words, if the public sector did not establish such policies, their hospitals would remain inefficient, merely guzzling funds, providing poor quality services. The public sector, with the funds coming from taxpayers will not be able to afford this scenario for too long, as evident in the near panic of many countries currently worn down by soaring healthcare costs. Thus, the earlier we recognize the implications of the scarcity of resources, a key underpinning of the motion of health services provision that we would be unable to stop, essentially, the sooner we would establish the appropriate policies to facilitate efficient functioning of government-run hospitals, if we indeed, must keep them. It is clear therefore that the present situation in many countries where government run health services is not sustainable, if these services did not match up to, or surpass those offered in the private sector, with which they would inevitably compete were governments to arrest the escalation in healthcare costs yet decline in services quality they face, these costs regardless. Besides being a recipe for a vicious cycle of heightening disease burden, hence more costs and spending, with potential devastating consequences for their economies, tarrying when we would still need to address these issues appropriately, as would increasingly become evident, makes no sense. This means then the inevitable realization of the reverse situation. Thus, would evolve from the natural tendency to swell public coffers these hospitals not just running more efficiently, hence not being competitive with private-sector hospitals, such policies as would give public sector workers options to attend private hospitals on the one hand, obviating the need so to do, on the other, but in fact, extracting clients from the private sector. In other words, whatever government hospital remains would be because they are more efficient and cost-effective. This scenario would inevitably lead to fusion, a collaborative tendency between public and private sector hospitals to exploit scale and scope economies for their mutual benefits. We thus not only see the possible direction of the evolution of employer-based health insurance, but also a situation wherein some of the public sector hospitals would die a natural death, literally, others absolved into larger enterprises both public and private, the whole concept of health services provision, brand new. We here use the term 'hospital' in a generic sense to refer to a unit of health service provision, although the concept of such a unit is also going to be fluid, as that of health service provision in general evolves. The point here then underscores the permanence rather than transience of employer-based health insurance, although as we have seen, the concept of the employer is also generic. These issues highlight the need for a thorough analysis for example, of the current controversy in the U.S regarding physician-owned and non-physician owned specialty hospitals, in response to which in fact legislators at both the state and federal levels want legislation that would ban physician ownership of hospitals[14, 15]. A recent study published on hospital characteristics and patient populations served by physician owned and non-physician owned orthopaedic specialty hospitals, underscores this point[16]. The researchers carried out a descriptive study using Medicare data of beneficiaries that had total hip replacement (THR) (N=10,478) and total knee replacement (TKR) (N=15,312) in 29 physician owned and 8 non physician owned specialty orthopaedic hospitals between 1999 and 2003 comparing hospital characteristics of physician owned and non-physician owned specialty hospitals. These included procedural volumes of major joint replacements (THR and TKR), hospital teaching status, and for profit status. They also compared demographics and prevalence of common co-morbid conditions for patients treated in both settings, and examined differences or otherwise in the socio-demographic characteristics of their neighbourhoods suing zip code level d ata. The study showed that physician owned specialty hospitals performed fewer major joint replacements on Medicare beneficiaries in 2003 than non-physician owed specialty hospitals (64 vs. 678, P<.001), were less likely to have links with a medical school (6% vs. 43%, P=.05), and likelier to be for profit (94% vs. 28%, P=.001). It also showed that patients who had major joint replacement in physician owned specialty hospitals were unlikelier to be black than patients in non-physician owned specialty hospitals (2.5% vs. 3.1% for THR, P=.15; 1.8% vs. 6.3% for TKR, P<.001), despite that physician owned specialty hospitals were in areas with more black residents (8.2% vs. 6.7%, P=.76). Additionally, the study showed that patients in physician owned hospitals had less incidents of most common comorbid illnesses such as heart failure and obesity (P<.05 for both). That the researchers concluded that physician owned specialty orthopaedic hospitals are significantly different from non-physician owned specialty orthopaedic hospitals hence may need the added scrutiny legislators proposed is, however, debatable, given our discussion thus far regarding the nature and scope of the government and indeed, the legislature, in health services provision. To start with, where would we place our wager on such legislation as proposed in the U.S given the almost commonsensical idea that the more of a particular surgical procedure a surgeon does, the more adept he or she becomes at it, which has led for to calls for regionalization of services in countries such as the UK? In other words, is the emergence of specialty hospitals centred on limited procedural aspects of medical practice such as cardiology, obstetrics and gynaecology or orthopaedics, such a bad thing, after all? Even if specialty hospitals preferentially admit low-risk patients than competing general hospitals, without showing benefits in risk-adjusted outcomes as their critics maintain17, which research confirms, is that in addition, also confirmed, that they seem to have 10%-20% lower risk-adjusted rates of adverse outcomes18, not antithetical to banning them? Should we not allow market forces to modulate the potential tendency of supplier-induced demand in physician-owned specialty hospitals, with service overutilization19, hence increased costs, which speaks to the need to rectify the pervasive information asymmetry in the health sector, instead of a wanton proscription of these hospitals? The point in fact is that the healthcare consumer would go to the general hospitals were they also delivering the high-quality services that specialty hospitals deliver, and at comparable prices, which would obviate the need for concerns regarding stratification, or service overutilization, equipped with the appropriate information to make such choices. In other words, and as noted earlier, we should promote the culture of efficiency among service providers, be it in the private or public sector. Thus, even among specialty hospitals, whether physician-owned or non-physician-owned, it is the ability to deliver efficient and cost-effective services that would determine, given free-market operations, which survives or becomes extinct. It is important to note that under those circumstances, it matters little, if at all, physician-owned hospitals choose not to provide services to people in whose neighbourhoods they are in, as competition would determine if they would remain there in the first place and for how much longer. In other words, why would even some of their clients not patronize a general hospital nearby that runs equally efficiently, and provides similar services at comparable if not even cheaper prices? In other words, perhaps such general hospitals have developed ways to ensure that high-risk patients become low-risk patients, other than excluding them from their practices. In other words, by improving outcomes, in addition to the attributes buoying competitiveness mentioned earlier, would such general hospitals not stand a better chance than the specialty hospitals, physician-owned or otherwise? Employers would be asking similar questions in the future in choosing to which health services providers to subscribe. The answers to the questions would also inform policy in the public and private sector, as both struggle, to balance the need and requirements for survival with those for health services provision to their workers. here is no doubt therefore that the emergence of specialty hospitals is in keeping with the inevitability of health services evolution along the directions of strengthening rather than weakening employer-based health insurance that essentially our thesis here. The deadlock in the recent negotiations in the U.S between General Motors Corp. (GM) and the United Auto Workers (UAW), which at some point led to workers picketing for a few days, highlights the intensity of some of the issues involved in health services provision for workers. In particular, how much the firm should deposit in its retirees' health care fund, the so-called Voluntary Employees Beneficiary Association, or VEBA, which UAW would manage, is the sticky point, literally in the current negotiations. GM currently has about $51 billion in unfunded retiree health care costs, all of which it is not under any compulsion to put into the VEBA, the disagreement being over how much GM should put in VEBA, and how much it pays in cash or stock20. GM has about 339,000 UAW retirees and spouses, and reportedly seeks to pay the union to form the VEBA to remove the health care liabilities from its accounts the UAW on the other hand, seeks assurances of new vehicles built in U.S. plants, in other words, job security, in return. The latter expects Ford Motor Co. and Chrysler LLC, the other two auto giants in Detroit, to match many of the terms of GM's deal. These negotiations also highlight the interdependence of workers and their employers that would feature increasingly prominently in the dynamics of their relations, and in particular regarding health services provision, in the years ahead. The question of the way it would play out is moot given not only that intrinsically, it connotes symbiosis, at least until these auto companies, are able to manufacture their vehicles exclusively by automation, applicable to all firms that need human capital, hence collaboration, to which that the strike action called by the UAW lasted only a few days, attests. It is the continued existence of this symbiotic dyad that would not only ensure that employer-sponsored survives, but indeed, thrives, but also dictates the approaches to ensuring it does as it maneuvers in the fluidity change impels in the health and related industries. In other words, employers, as noted earlier, would be keen to ask questions and seek answers to such as those noted above regarding specialty hospitals, for example. Indeed, part of the corporate health strategy of discerning firms would in future be to infuse the answers to such questions in their conceptualization of and approaches to negotiations regarding healthcare with their workers. The answers to such questions for examples could help determine how much firms pay out and in what forms, and indeed, what employers do with the money, the nature and amount of stocks offered employers for example tied to acquiescence to and participation in health promotion initiatives. Clearly, such initiatives would not only benefit the individual but also create opportunities for long-term enhanced productivity that on the aggregate would contribute positively to the company's bottom line. In other words, firms would increasingly need to be conversant with developments in the health sector, and in related domains and incorporate some of these developments into their strategic framework. These developments might be local or national, or even concern events happening internationally, for example, the measures employed in a plant in another country were there a sudden outbreak of, say, avian flu, and those taken even prior to it. Thus, rather than mandate vaccination for all staff, for example, to prevent a particular disease, a firm could tie such vaccination to a reward, for example, in stocks, or bonuses. It could offer to pay 50% of the costs of a treadmill, or some other fitness/exercise equipment, for its workers, or offer free online courses or even workshops on health and fitness for its workers, attendance at which attracts some sort of reward, say 'health points' tied to year-end bonuses, which those that did not attend will not receive. Firms would also increasingly emphasize a 'corporate culture' of ownership, inherent anyway in the symbiosis, but which would require re-emphasizing from time to time, toremind all, workers and employers alike, of the need to remain healthy in the overall interests of both parties. This would cultivate a voluntary adherence to sound health principles from which both parties would benefit tremendously. In other words, there would be no need to compel anyone to stay healthy were we to recognize the potential for an understanding of the stakes that we, in general have, as humans, and which we could impart on our relatives and friends who might lack the wherewithal, intellectual or otherwise, so to do. Firms would therefore be curtailing healthcare expenditures on their workers and relatives also focusing on rectifying the information asymmetry that typically hinders such understanding. Such an endeavour would also not just be helping rational decision-making regarding the choice of healthcare providers, and in optimizing service utilization, but also in promoting the cultivation of healthy lifestyles, and in disease prevention. Thus would evolve an appreciation in full of the fundamental underpinnings mentioned above, for example, freedom from coercion, of the motion of healthcare delivery that makes it inevitable for the perpetuity of employer-sponsored health insurance. Given this tendency therefore, would also be, and as a consequence, the diffusion of such understanding into other spheres of our affairs, in tandem. It would become clear that the employer/employee dyadic is a fundamental association upon which the survival of society indeed, predicates, which would make measures, legislative or otherwise that purports to terminate that association potentially antithetical to our very existence. That the association is voluntary is exigent on the need to ensure its survival, if not indeed, imperative, would be what to which the outcome of that exigency appropriately amounts. The evolution of the success of the China economy is a case in point. The economic reforms in that country would eventually turn into political reforms that would increasingly ensure the sustainability of that success, given that it is unlikely to do otherwise, as it transitions into global economic spotlight, besides the dramatic improvement in its peoples' wellbeing. Thus, the economic gains that have accrued due to the country embracing free-market operations would dissolve into nothingness over time, if it failed to embrace the individual's liberty. Indeed, even in those countries embrace the liberty of the individual, mandating one thing or another, including healthcare runs counter to the freedom to choose that is essential to the realization of the benefits accruable to the full expression of the fundamentals on which the inevitable evolution of the progress of humankind predicates. Thus, it would be futile to mandate health insurance when this would not make some purchase it anyway, for whatever reason, perhaps even simply because of the mandate. The frustration of some policy makers keen to curtail the soaring health expenditures of their jurisdictions in proposing such mandates in one form or another is understandable. What is often not, is their seeming inability, if not even refusal, to see the bigger picture, literally, and to appreciate that such mandates would unlikely work, and could end up being counterproductive to their stated goals. A crucial aspect of the need for freedom in the association mentioned above between workers and their employers is the desire that would evolve matters handled appropriately by the firms and employers, or their unions, on the parts of both, to ensure the sustainability of their firm. This emphasizes the resulting sense of ownership that would engender voluntary compliance with initiatives that would secure this sustainability, which coercion is unlikely to achieve, hence which firms would no doubt increasingly, de-emphasize in their healthcare strategies. Imagine therefore the consequences for morbidity and mortality, healthcare costs, hence spending, of the shunning say an individual mandate to purchase health insurance by some, as for a firm, any measures that suggest coercion, rather than collaboration in their approaches to healthcare. It is thus unlikely that it would take very long for the proponents of such individual health insurance mandates or any attempt to legislate healthcare to realize that this is just compromising progress, in particular, as the adoption of approaches to healthcare that emphasize on the contrary the need to engage rather than coerce individuals is inevitable, ultimately. The point is that it is important to recognize that not only is employer-sponsored health insurance potentially capable of solving many of the problems that plague many health systems, for example, the lack of health insurance by a large number of persons in some countries, but also prevent some new ones emerging.

Firms would increasingly realize that their healthcare strategies could either enhance the much company loyalty that they so covet, but which are increasingly hard to find, or further dampen. New technologies, swift capital flow and labor, and globalization, among others, make corporate organizational flux the stark reality that many would claim compromise the ability of organizations to ensure this loyalty, and indeed, makes it necessary for them to seek new ways to cement the worker/employer association. It is also increasingly evident that workers are more mobile, engage in multiple careers in their working lives, and acknowledge the dissolution of the borders, organizational, national, and otherwise that hitherto seemed impenetrable. Thus, firms would need to appreciate increasingly the evolution of the worker/ employer relationship, and the changes that it impels to develop innovative ways to secure the sense of ownership that comes with loyalty crucial to the continuity of the dyad. Rather than predicate it on coercion, they would need to do so on voluntary collaboration, encouraged via meaningful incentives that would not create dissent among employees, or between them and their employers, but would rather inculcate in the workforce, an innovative bent. Thus, workers and their employers would benefit from the mutual respect that such an approach engenders, forging trust and commitment, albeit for the time the association lasts, sufficient for those coming into the association anew to build upon, the recipe the firms needs to guarantee not only its survival, but its profitability. Finding a common ground on health issues is thus crucial between employers and workers, and underscores the importance of employer-sponsored health insurance, and the need for firms to attend to it as it evolves, and to make it work. Corporate success would increasingly predicate on the effective management of the employer/employee dyad, which as we noted earlier, would be ever more fluid due to the dissolution of the erstwhile barriers that form a cocoon round the dyad, creating a sense of security in both parties, albeit rooted in assumptions within a coercive context. With workers increasingly mobile, for example, they would no longer have to operate blindly within stipulated company rules and regulations, some of which essentially strip them of at least part of their identity. New formulas would have to emerge to ensure recruitment and retention, and the fortunes of firms would increasingly depend on their management being able to develop innovative ideas to cultivate corporate culture and company loyalty in an ever-changing dispensation. Firms would thus need to pay more attention to their healthcare strategies, as this is not only fundamentally crucial to the survival of the dyad, hence of the firms, but also as it touches on the core human tendency to survive, and the means to ensure it does. It would become evident more and more that supporting this endeavour would likely promote the trust between employers and employees, germane to the sense of ownership that fosters the voluntary collaboration on healthcare initiatives, among others, blossoming. This sense of ownership engenders commitment, which in turn, boosts productivity, not just in facilitating the entrenchment of a healthy workforce, but also in nurturing creativity, hence innovation, crucial elements of competitiveness that firms would need even more in an increasingly globalized economy. Each firm would need to align the aspirations of its workers with its corporate goals in ways that would be mutually beneficial to both. By focusing on healthcare and establishing the appropriate strategies to ensure its provision to its workers at affordable costs, the firm would be facilitating this alignment. It is thus clear the role that healthcare would play in the future of firms hence the importance that they would likely accord it in their corporate affairs. That they would not just see healthcare within the corporate context but as an integral aspect of the place of their organizations in the overall economic scheme in their jurisdictions would further be catalytic in their quest to ensure the alignment. Thus, and as we noted earlier, employer-sponsored healthcare would be central to any health system, and indeed, would be direction that health systems would, inevitably head, given its key role in this scheme. The results of a recent study that showed that firms could reduce absenteeism and boost workers' health investing in depressed employees, promptly providing them treatment and even offering them telephone psychotherapy, for examples21 is instructive in this regard. Indeed, one of the researchers Dr. Philip Wang of the National Institute of Mental Health, which funded the study, published in the Journal of the American Medical Association observed that firms that spend money on depression are simply being prudent, as employees that received such intensive intervention worked averagely about two weeks more than those who received the usual care. The latter approach, merely advising the worker to visit his or her doctor or a mental health specialist, thus is not enough as additionally, more workers in the intervention group remained in employment at the end of the year, the duration of the study. More precisely, 93 percent did, compared with 88 percent, in the group that received usual care, providing employers, savings that reduced hiring and training costs, noted the researchers, and employees in the intervention group were about 40 percent likelier to recover from depression 21. Indeed, preliminary results from the study indicate savings from more hours the intervention employers worked averaged to about $1,800 per employee, much more than the program's initial cost of $100 to $400 per worker, the benefits also likely more than other costs, for examples, medications, noted the researchers. With depression common in the workplace in the country, about 6 percent of employees annually affected, with a cost of more than $30 billion annually in lost productivity, as co-author Ronald Kessler, a Harvard Medical School researcher, noted, employers would no doubt be keen to apply the findings in this study to their organizations. Six hundred and four white-collar and blue-collar workers at 16 large U.S. firms participated in the study, janitors, pilots, bankers, truckers, and lawyers, included, 50% on usual care, including a letter prompting those depressed to contact their primary-care doctor or call United Behavioural Health (UBH), a large managed-care company involved in the study, for referral to a psychiatrist. Those in the intervention group had repeated telephone calls during non-work hours from UBH case managers trained in mental health treatment urging employees to receive treatment, even making follow-up calls from time to time to see how it was proceeding21. In fact, employers that shunned help received offers from case managers of telephone psychotherapy, which many workers considered less stigmatizing and more convenient than going to see a psychiatrist, 60% of those in the intervention group likelier to receive treatment from a psychiatrist, although 40% of employees in both groups received antidepressants. Employers would no doubt pay increasing attention to studies such as this one, which buttress the points made here that employer-sponsored health insurance, given its benefits to both employers and workers, and indeed, to the overall economy, would not only survive but would play an increasingly pivotal role in healthcare delivery in the years ahead.

References:

1. Available at: http://www.latimes.com/news/local/la-me-health23aug23,0,7082425.story?coll=la-home-center Accessed on August 24, 2007

2. Hacker, JS. Healing Our Sicko Health Care System. N Engl J Med. 2007 Aug 23; 357(8):733-5.

3. Consumer Reports health insurance survey reveals 1 in 4 people insured but not adequately covered. Washington, DC: Consumers Union, 2007.

4. Himmelstein DU, Warren E, Thorne D, Woolhandler S. Illness and injury as contributors to bankruptcy. Health Aff (Millwood) 2005;:W5-63.

5. Blendon RJ, Schoen C, DesRoches CM, Osborn R, Scoles KL, Zapert K. Inequities in health care: a five-country survey. Health Aff (Millwood) 2002; 21:182-191.

6. Available at: http://www.usatoday.com/news/washington/2005-03-16- medicare-riddle_x.htm Accessed on August 24, 2007

7. Hacker, JS. Health care for America: a proposal for guaranteed, affordable health care for all Americans building on Medicare and employment-based

insurance. Briefing paper, Washington, DC: Economic Policy Institute, January 11, 2007. Available at: http://www.sharedprosperity.org/bp180.html. Accessed August 24, 2007

8. Available at:

http://www.census.gov/hhes/www/hlthins/hlthin06/hlth06asc.html Accessed on August 29, 2007

9. Available at: http://www.courant.com/business/hc-mercer0906.artsep06,0,949750.story Accessed on September 10, 2007

10. Available at: http://www.post-gazette.com/pg/06324/739384-28.stm Accessed on September 10, 2007.

11. Available at:

http://www.kaisernetwork.org/daily_reports/rep_index.cfm?hint=3&DR_ID=4 1163Accessed on September 10, 2007

12. Available at: http://www.ama-

assn.org/amednews/2007/10/01/gvl11001.htm Accessed on September 24,

2007.

13. Available at:

http://news.yahoo.com/s/ap/20070917/ap_on_el_pr/clinton_health_care&pri

nter=1;_ylt=AoUVMXBhcbwqgY.50ZLEnWRh24cA Accessed on September 24, 2007.

14. Medicare Prescription Drug Improvement and Modernization Act of 2003, 108-173.

15. Missouri Hospital Association. Missouri Hospital Association Information for the Missouri Senate Committee on Certificate of Need. Available at: http://aaasc.org/state/documents/MOHospAssn.08.01.06.pdf#search=%22what%20states%20ban%20physician%20owned%20specialty%20hospitals%22: Accessed September 29, 2007

16. Cram P, Vaughan-Sarrazin MS, Rosenthal GE. Hospital characteristics and patient populations served by physician owned and non-physician owned orthopedic specialty hospitals. BMC Health Services Research 2007, 7:155 (25 September 2007)

17. Casalino LP, Devers KJ, Brewster LR. Focused Factories? Physician-Owned Specialty Facilities. Health Aff. 2003; 22(6):56-67.

18. Cram P, Rosenthal GE, Vaughan-Sarrazin MS. Cardiac revascularization in specialty and general hospitals. N Engl J Med. 2005; 352(14):1454-62.

19. De Jaegher K, Jegers M. The physician-patient relationship as a game of strategic information transmission. Health Economics. 2001; 10(7):651-68.

20. Available at:

http://biz.yahoo.com/ap/070923/auto_talks.html?.v=11&printer=1 accessed on September 29, 2007

Conclusion

The increased awareness of the public in many countries regarding health issues speaks to the recognition of the importance of health not just for the individual but also for society. It is also reassuring in that it signifies the potential of the concerted efforts required to improve health services to work, with interests by all stakeholders in health matters ever heightening. For too long, and despite the obvious implications of ill health for economic productivity and societal progress, both individuals and the sources from which they receive healthcare, be they from their employers in the public or the private sector, have not shown the sort of vigour in addressing the problems that compromise healthcare delivery. As a result, the problems continue to worsen, adding substantially to the burden of diseases for all.

Only recently, with research findings on safety issues in health services provision, and the soaring costs of healthcare, publicized in the media, have attitudes towards health issues started to change significantly, with healthcare consumers and other stakeholders asking serious questions regarding their health services, and healthcare delivery in general. Even then, given the increasing rates of overweight and obesity for examples, it is doubtful the extent to which this increasing exposure of the public to progress in medical knowledge, including our understanding of diseases appear to been making a difference to peoples' attitudes regarding their health and lifestyles.

In other words, it is no longer a matter of people being unaware of the dangers of excessive weight, or what they could do to curb it, but whether they feel concerned enough to do so, and even if so, willing to give up their old habits and adopt healthier lifestyles. This leaves one wondering though what it takes to make people adopt healthier lifestyles, for example quit smoking, given the surfeit of information out there, including on the Internet, not to mention government efforts in many countries to reduce smoking rates by banning smoking in public and certain other places. Are people just simply suicidal, perhaps without their knowing, or we have not understood well enough some of the roots of these behaviours?

The questions one could ask are legion, as are the potential answers, were we to attempt to start with, to understand these issues, perhaps likely frustrating a situation, and likely to demoralize all but the zealous, some would insist, but which it should be quite easy to see, we would have to do anyway, for our collective interests. In other words, we need not quibble, as currently in the U.S., over the State Children's Health Insurance Program (SCHIP), a national program Senator Ted Kennedy and First Lady (now a senator from New York) Hillary Rodham Clinton originated in 1997 to provide, health insurance for families overqualified for Medicaid, but not earning enough to afford private insurance. Rather we should examine how such children would receive coverage as members of a family earning an income, regardless of where the income is coming from, even if welfare, with the choice to receive health services where they choose, in the free market.

That the U.S., Congress passed a bill recently to expand SCHIP from $5 billion annually to $35 billion over five years, but the bill later vetoed by President Bush on October 03, 2007, and that in spite of SCHIP, the number of uninsured children keeps increasing, are instructive, given that it is unlikely that the president hates children. They are also perhaps indicative of the chances of mismanagement of the program that characterize governments' involvement in what indeed, should operate in the free markets, which we need to look into. The debate on SCHIP incidentally is ongoing and would likely persist in the political arena, although there is probably no doubt in the minds of all involved in the debate, what the future portends for government involvement in health services provision.

As we have here argued, we would simply continue to grope being inflexible about entrenched attitudes, the costs of tarrying to make the required changes to our conceptualization of health and healthcare delivery, only likely to heighten the same angst that make us shudder to remove healthcare coverage for millions of American children. We should remember though that in doing so, we would be providing healthcare to these children more appropriately. What sense does it make not being able to provide healthcare to even a million children because we cannot just find the money? Whereas, we would be able to continue to provide not just children, but to all, with qualitative and affordable healthcare if we were not driven by, perhaps even political hubris.

We envisage that in reading this book, the reader would have been able to detect the message that we need to wake up literally to the urgent issues that confront us regarding health services provision, and stop gerrymandering with health issues. The costs of delaying action are simply too high especially given that we would still have to come back to take those actions were we to move our health systems forward. The approaches to addressing healthcare issues would indeed vary in different health jurisdictions, but there are commonalities that we need to recognize, that of the pivotal roles that employer-sponsored health insurance would play in health systems worldwide being the centerpiece of our discussions in this book, as is the potential means to actualizing these roles by firms, small and large.

The health of workers and their families, including children, should be the legitimate concern of their employers, considering the symbiotic dyad that the employee/employer relationship constitutes. However, it should primarily be that of the worker and his or her family. As we have here noted, the potential for an arrangement between workers and their employers that would enable the realization of what we termed the dual healthcare delivery objectives (DHDO) is real, details of which arrangement would constitute some of the more specific aspects of the healthcare delivery enterprise. However, since both elements of the dyad have a stake in the achievement of the DHDO, the prospects of this happening increase significantly, as opposed to government providing the services in which latter case, the incentive for competitiveness is lacking given that the funds for providing the services come from public coffers.

Thus, and as we have here stressed, firms need to acknowledge the facts of the situation in which they are, relative to other aspects of the economy in which they operate. In other words, it is not a matter of imposition by society on them to provide health services for their workers, as in some sort of government mandate, but rather it is inherent in the very nature of business and of society for them, and not government to play this role. That individuals simply must accept responsibilities for their actions as much as every one else must, enhances the likelihood of the arrangement between workers and their employers that coincide and that both need working, handled appropriately, which indeed, is in the interests of both parties, as we have seen in our discussion here, to do. This scenario would likely play out in ways that an expectation of convergence of interests yielding projected outcomes would be eminently justified.

Our emphasis in this book besides highlighting the aforementioned, what we could term the theoretical underpinnings of our position on the crucial role that employers would play in healthcare delivery in the years ahead, is also about firms making the best use of the opportunities their acquiescence to their roles in the health systems in their jurisdictions present. Additionally, perhaps, more than being prepared to tackle the challenges too, we also stress the need for these firms actually to turn them as much as possible into new prospects that would enhance their chances of achieving their stated health services provision goals. Here again, we see how the workings of the activities of the firms actualizing their healthcare strategic objectives could in addition to enabling them achieve the dual healthcare delivery objectives, in point of fact also create opportunities for them to gain competitive edge in their industry.

This book therefore presents a perspective on health and healthcare delivery that based on the fundamental ideals of freedom, democracy, and free market operations, reveals the profound roots of human behaviour that belie many of the actions that we take for granted, and their imperfections. These flaws in our behaviours are evident in the problems that confront our health systems, themselves, manifest of the need to revisit these fundamental ideals that we have not in fact apparently committed to optimally, and in some countries, not at all. In other words, we need to create innovative enabling milieus for these ideals to manifest, as they should within the prevailing circumstances. Thus, health systems management has moved on from half a century ago, for example in the U.S., when the "New Deal" operated essentially in tandem with the vision of industry, in particular the major automakers, deals with workers' union emergent now out of sync with contemporary realities, yet have spawned an entire industry, today's health plans, its relic.

As we have here noted, workers and their employers still need to work out amicable deals, only that the framework for such deals must situate in the C21st. In pursuing the fundamental ideals therefore, we must factor in contemporary realities, and project as far as we could into the future. These ideals would still guide the nature of the contract between workers and their employers except that both would 'own' the contract, and not view it as an instrument to achieve exclusively, focused stakes. In fact, workers, and their employers would need to start to view their interests as coinciding, which the cultivation of trust between both, would engender. Such a scenario would offer both the enabling milieu for the ideals mentioned earlier to flourish. In effect, healthcare would forge collaboration between workers and their employees conceptualized appropriately, as we have here counselled.

It is clear therefore, the basis of our contention that employer-based health insurance would reign supreme, literally in the healthcare delivery scheme in the years ahead. This puts the onus on firms to ensure that they are equipped adequately not just to play the role expected of them, but also to garner competitive advantage in implementing their innovative healthcare strategies. We dare say in fact that the approaches by firms to developing their healthcare strategies, the initiatives that emerge thereof, the manner of their implementation, and their success or otherwise would be defining characteristics, among others, of business success in the future. There should not be in fact, thus, any reason for firms to discountenance the pull that the opportunities their healthcare strategies would present, given that these could only translate to a further boost in their bottom line, handled appropriately. his last statement refers in particular to the potential for these strategies to warrant investments, sometimes significantly, in healthcare information and communications technologies (healthcare IVT) for example. Because the benefits in particular in material terms derivable from such investments might initially be cryptic, not only might management be unable to justify and secure funding for the technologies, but it might not in fact even consider implementing them at all. Yet, the technologies, long-term, might confer such benefits in human, and indeed, in pecuniary terms in savings in health spending that might outweigh the costs involved in implementing them. This underscores the need for firms to adopt flexible, short-and long-range approaches to their healthcare strategies as crucial aspects of ensuring that these strategies deliver on their promise.

The dimensions that would warrant considerations by firms committed to embracing the principles here elucidated would therefore be many, even complex. However, this is in keeping with the complexity that change in our increasingly hyper-competitive global economy prescribes. Indeed, in attuning to complexity, we might be able to devise simplicity, for example, a digest of research materials, which might make healthcare initiatives easier to implement, and which emphasizes the leadership role that firms would need to play in ensuring the success of the employer/employee dyad. No doubt, each member of the dyad would need to play its part, but leadership would need to come from the firm, in whose charge the resources for health services provision, essentially reside. This, however, does not mean that the firms should lord it over their workers, and in fact, they should remember that they need to promote trust among their workers, which coercion, would unlikely achieve.

As we also noted in our discussions in the book, it might not be easy for firms to embrace many of the ideas in this book, in particular given the current state of affairs, around which, they would likely imagine they need to organize their finances. It is not difficult for example to see why small firms, and indeed, large firms are having difficult in the U.S., meeting their health benefits obligations to their workers. The question is though if they would rather not, as many of the smaller firms, are in fact already doing, provide their workers with healthcare coverage. Even if it seemed prudent not to do so in the short term, which is unlikely going to be the case, it would certainly not be a good idea in the long term denying their workers such coverage.

This is so given not only the chances of the workers being unhealthy, which would compromise their productivity, and encourage absenteeism, or even 'presenteeism,' as we have discussed in this book, but also of some actually leaving the firms to work elsewhere. This, depending on how critical their services are, and how easy replacing them is, could spell doom, literally, for the firms, indeed, even in the short term. These issues underscore why in fact, it is important that firms come to terms with this rather crucial role that they need to play in their workers' healthcare provision, and work towards playing the role effectively, for the sake of both parties. No matter how hard therefore it is for firms to acquiesce to these roles, that they would also benefit from playing them effectively should spur them into taking the appropriate actions toward actualizing the roles.

It is also important to emphasize that firms would need the support of other healthcare stakeholders to embrace their roles in the health systems in the jurisdictions in which they operate. One cannot gainsay that government regulations could jeopardize their efforts in this regard. So could lack of cooperation by certain industries that might feel threatened by the initiatives taken by firms regarding health services provision for their workers and in general to achieve the dual healthcare delivery objectives. There are indeed, many ways the efforts of firms could come to naught, and it would take not just these efforts applied unilaterally, but also in collaboration with others, and not just their workers but also other stakeholders for the firms to achieve the desire success.

It is also important to emphasize that the support of other healthcare stakeholders would be crucial for firms to embrace their roles in the health systems in the jurisdictions in which they operate. One cannot gainsay that government regulations could jeopardize their efforts in this regard. So could lack of cooperation by certain industries that might feel threatened by the initiatives taken by firms regarding health services provision for their workers and in general to achieve the dual healthcare delivery objectives. There are indeed, many ways the efforts of firms could come to naught, and it would take not just these efforts applied unilaterally, but also in collaboration with others, and not just their workers but also other stakeholders for the firms to achieve the desire success.

Ultimately, the cooperation by all stakeholders would be crucial to employer-sponsored health insurance securing its central place in the healthcare delivery scheme. However, as plausible as it might seem, at first that firms would need to cajole, essentially, others into teaming up with them to achieve the goals of qualitative, and affordable health services provision to workers, it would soon become apparent that all healthcare stakeholders indeed, have a stake in the matter. It is thus, likely not going to require much effort on the firms' part after all to get others on the team. In fact, it underscores why the content of this book would be invaluable material for not just firms, but also all healthcare stakeholders. As firms would, in the main, ultimately, other stakeholders would also recognize the need for us all to be determined to not just address, but also in fact solve the problems that plague health systems currently. It would become evident that we could not achieve this goal being inflexible and sticking to 'business as usual' in our approaches to healthcare delivery. We would acknowledge the need for these approaches to be consonant with developments in medicine and technology for examples, and indeed, other relevant domains to work. We would start to appreciate the significance of change and the need for us to adapt to change and most of all, we would recognize that employer-sponsored health insurance is pivotal our prospects of achieving our desired objectives, and in moving our health systems forward.

Indeed, this book, would have achieved its stated objectives were it to influence the outlook of these stakeholders to health and healthcare delivery issues, crucial elements of the success of our sojourn as humans through life.

Thank you, for your interest in traveling with us this far.

Copyright Bankix Systems Ltd October 9, 2007

www.ingramcontent.com/pod-product-compliance
Lightning Source LLC
Chambersburg PA
CBHW030654220526
45463CB00005B/1769